The second edition of the *ABC of Resuscitation* incorporates the latest standards and guidelines for cardiopulmonary resuscitation issued by the Resuscitation Council (UK) in 1989. There are three new chapters – one on trauma, one on resuscitation in late pregnancy, and one on avoiding HIV infection – and throughout, recommendations have been updated where necessary and other revisions have been made in view of current theory and practice. Written by members of the Resuscitation Council (UK) and other invited experts, the new edition of *ABC of Resuscitation* offers the most up to date information and advice on this vital aspect of health care.

ABC OF RESUSCITATION

ABC OF
RESUSCITATION

edited by

T R EVANS FRCP

Consultant cardiologist,
Royal Free Hospital, London

on behalf of
the Resuscitation Council (UK)
with contributions from the
following members of the Resuscitation Council

PETER J F BASKETT, A JOHN CAMM, DOUGLAS
CHAMBERLAIN, T R EVANS, JUDITH FISHER, MARK HARRIES,
ALASTAIR McGOWAN, ANDREW K MARSDEN, A D MILNER,
A D REDMOND, R S SIMONS, BRIAN STEGGLES,
RICHARD VINCENT, DAVID A ZIDEMAN

and additional contributions from
T HILARY HOWELLS, G A D REES, B A WILLIS,
GERALYN WYNNE

Published by the British Medical Journal,
Tavistock Square, London WC1H 9JR

Acknowledgment

Ambu International Ltd, Laerdal Medical Ltd, and Vitalo-graph Ltd kindly provided photographs of their equipment.

© British Medical Journal 1990

First edition 1986
Second impression 1988
Third impression 1988
Fourth impression 1989
Second edition 1990

British Library Cataloguing in Publication Data

ABC of resuscitation—2nd ed.
1. Man. Resuscitation
I. Evans, T.R.
615.8′043

ISBN 0–7279–0260–1

Typeset and printed by Latimer Trend & Company Ltd,
Plymouth, Great Britian.

Contents

Page

Introduction ix

Recognising a cardiac arrest and providing basic life support JUDITH M FISHER, *general practitioner, Chingford, London E4 9SY, and chairman of the British Association of Immediate Care* 1

Ventricular fibrillation DOUGLAS CHAMBERLAIN, *consultant cardiologist, Royal Sussex County Hospital, Brighton BN3 5BE* 5

Asystole and electromechanical dissociation A JOHN CAMM, *professor of clinical cardiology, St George's Hospital Medical School, London SW17 0QT* 9

The airway at risk ROBERT S SIMONS, *consultant anaesthetist, and* T HILARY HOWELLS, *director of department of anaesthesia, Royal Free Hospital, London NW3 2QG* 12

Advanced life support in general practice BRIAN STEGGLES, *general practitioner, Tavistock, Devon* 17

Resuscitation by ambulance crews RICHARD VINCENT, *consultant cardiologist, Brighton Health District* 21

Resuscitation in the accident and emergency department ANDREW K MARSDEN, *consultant in emergency medicine, and* ALASTAIR MCGOWAN, *consultant in emergency medicine, Pinderfields General Hospital, Wakefield WF1 4DG* 26

Resuscitation of multiply injured patients ANDREW K MARSDEN. 30

Resuscitation in hospital T R EVANS, *consultant cardiologist, Royal Free Hospital, London NW3 2QG* 34

Postresuscitation care A D REDMOND, *consultant in accident and emergency medicine, University Hospital of South Manchester, Manchester M20 8LR* 37

Training and retention of skills GERALYN WYNNE, *resuscitation training officer, Royal Free Hospital, London NW3 2QG* 40

Training manikins ROBERT S SIMONS, *consultant anaesthetist, Royal Free Hospital, London NW3 2QG* 45

Resuscitation in pregnancy G A D REES, *consultant anaesthetist, and* B A WILLIS, *locum consultant anaesthetist, University Hospital of Wales, Cardiff* 50

Resuscitation at birth A D MILNER, *professor of paediatric respiratory medicine, University Hospital, Nottingham* 54

Resuscitation of infants and children DAVID A ZIDEMAN, *consultant anaesthetist and honorary senior lecturer, Royal Postgraduate Medical School, Hammersmith Hospital, London W12 0HS* 57

Drowning and near drowning MARK HARRIES, *consultant respiratory physician, Northwick Park Hospital, Harrow, Middlesex HA1 3AU* .. 62

AIDS, hepatitis, and resuscitation DAVID A ZIDEMAN 65

Ethics of resuscitation   PETER J F BASKETT, *consultant anaesthetist, Bristo*
   Royal Infirmary and Frenchay Hospital, Bristol   66

Further reading   68

Index   69

Introduction

In the 1950s the work of researchers such as Elam and Safar showed that expired air respiration, the so called "kiss of life" or "mouth to mouth respiration," was the most effective method of artificial respiration. Then in 1960 Jude, Kouwenhoven, and Knickerbocker published their classic work on closed chest cardiac compression, showing that circulation could be maintained without thoracotomy during cardiac arrest. About the same time closed chest defibrillation came into widespread use, making the resuscitation of patients in ventricular fibrillation a frequent occurrence.

It was realised that patients at a high risk of cardiac arrest should be nursed in units where prompt resuscitation, particularly by defibrillation, was available. Thus coronary units were established because many patients with acute myocardial infarction suffered a cardiac arrest, particularly in the early hours after the acute event. Moreover, necropsy studies had shown that many patients dying after an infarction had sustained only a small infarct and that their death was due to the rhythm disturbance—the concept of "the heart too good to die."

Once the place of hospital resuscitation had become established, attention turned to the fact that up to 60% of all patients who died after acute myocardial infarction did so before they reached hospital. It is believed that the first mobile intensive care units were operated in Russia, but in the West credit must be given to Pantridge in Belfast, who pioneered the first mobile coronary care units manned by a doctor and a nurse. Early experience in Belfast showed clearly that the incidence of arrhythmias immediately after acute myocardial infarction was very high, and many patients reached by his mobile units were resuscitated outside hospital and survived to be discharged home. The Pantridge group also drew attention to the fact that basic resuscitation carried out by bystanders before the mobile coronary care unit arrived was an important determinant of survival.

In Seattle Cobb has developed what is probably the most sophisticated community based resuscitation delivery system in the world. In the USA paramedics, highly trained emergency medical personnel, developed from the medical corpsmen in Vietnam. Doctors and nurses do not usually staff the emergency vehicles, but paramedics trained in basic and advanced life support race to the scene and provide resuscitation under the direction of emergency physicians. To reduce the time to the start of basic life support there has been an intensive programme of training citizens to perform cardiopulmonary resuscitation as well as telephone instructions given by the fire dispatcher receiving the emergency call to the person calling for help. Because the fire department in Seattle and adjacent King County operate emergency medical services, a tiered response is operated so that a standard fire engine with a crew races to the scene to start resuscitation, and this is followed by what would be a standard ambulance in the UK, although many of the emergency medical technicians carry and use defibrillators. The paramedic unit, which arrives within five to ten minutes of a call, should find cardiopulmonary resuscitation in progress and often defibrillation already attempted.

Seattle and King County researchers have shown clearly that the two important factors that determine whether a patient will survive a cardiac arrest from ventricular fibrillation outside hospital are (*a*) the time to the start of basic resuscitation and (*b*) the time to defibrillation. Intensive efforts have therefore been made to reduce both times to the minimum, with the result that up to 30% of patients who suffer ventricular fibrillation in that area of the USA survive to leave hospital.

In the United Kingdom we have been slower to improve community resuscitation, but following the lead of Belfast and more recently Brighton, the latter using ambulancemen trained in advanced resuscitation, progress is now being made. The advent of a nationwide programme of extended training of ambulance staff in resuscitation and the "Save a Life" campaign aimed at training the community in basic resuscitation via television programmes backed by local practical training are important milestones.

We must not forget that hospital staff often do not possess the skills even in basic resuscitation that might be expected. Alarmingly poor performances by house staff have been documented on several occasions and have led in many medical schools and hospitals to the improved training of medical students and junior doctors in basic and advanced cardiopulmonary resuscitation. On the general wards it is nearly always nursing staff who start resuscitation, and our studies at the Royal Free have shown poor performance by trained nursing staff in resuscitation, indicating the need for more time to be spent on training and revision of skills. Training alone is not enough—more research needs to be carried out to assess the best training methods, the best resuscitation manikins for practice, and how often revision is required.

The Resuscitation Council (UK) comprises doctors from many different specialist and general practice backgrounds who share a desire to improve the standard of resuscitation. The council has produced flow charts showing suggested algorithms for both basic and advanced life support techniques, together with a pocket flip chart and simple manual on basic life support. It has also initiated a multicentre survey of the results of resuscitation in the UK with the support initially of the Laerdal Foundation and later of the British Heart Foundation.

My colleagues on the Resuscitation Council and other invited experts have collaborated to produce this *ABC of Resuscitation*, which we now offer not as a manual or textbook but, we hope, as a useful guide to resuscitation for the late 1980s.

TOM EVANS
Vice Chairman
Resuscitation Council (UK)

Introduction to the second edition

The 2nd edition of the *ABC of Resuscitation* has been produced to follow the issue of the 1989 Resuscitation Council (UK) standards and guidelines for cardiopulmonary resuscitation.

Recommendations have been updated where necessary, and other revisions have been made in view of current theory and practice. There are three new chapters, one on trauma, one on resuscitation in late pregnancy, and one on HIV (human immunodeficiency virus) and other infections.

Since the last edition, the Royal College of Physicians of London has issued a very important report on training and organisation in resuscitation and a Joint Colleges Liaison Committee with the Ambulance Service has been set up. Also a European Resuscitation Council has recently been formed. There seems to be greatly increased awareness of the need for resuscitation training at all levels, and the requirement to show resuscitation skills in many professional examinations is welcomed, as is the new Diploma in Immediate Care of the College of Surgeons of Edinburgh.

I am grateful to Geralyn Wynne, district resuscitation training officer at the Royal Free Hospital and chairman of the Association of Resuscitation Training Officers, for her help in editing this revised ABC.

T R EVANS
Chairman
Resuscitation Council (UK)

RECOGNISING A CARDIAC ARREST AND PROVIDING BASIC LIFE SUPPORT

JUDITH M FISHER

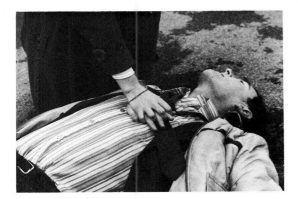

The combination of expired air respiration[1] and external chest compression[2] forms the basis of modern basic life support—cardiopulmonary resuscitation.[3]

The term "cardiac arrest" implies a sudden interruption of cardiac output, which may be reversible with appropriate treatment (cessation of heart activity as a terminal event in serious illness is thus excluded).

Initial assessment: approach, assess, and establish an airway

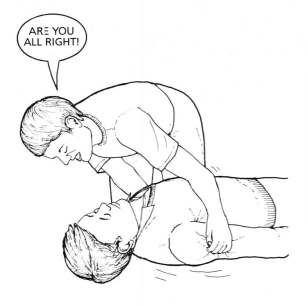

ARE YOU ALL RIGHT!

Resuscitation is the emergency treatment of any condition in which the brain fails to receive enough oxygen. The basic technique involves a rapid simple assessment of the patient, the ABC of resuscitation. A is for assess and airway, B is for breathing, and C is for circulation. Rapidly assess the danger to the casualty and you from such hazards as falling masonry, gas, electricity, fire, or traffic; there is no sense in having two casualties. Establish whether the patient is conscious by enquiring loudly "What has happened?" or "Are you alright?" while shaking him gently by the shoulder, being careful not to aggravate any existing injury, particularly of the cervical spine. At the same time (and at regular intervals throughout the resuscitation attempt if there is no initial response) shout for help.

Airway

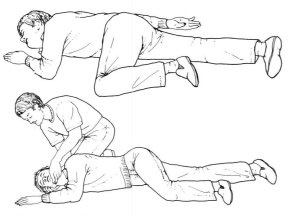

Recovery position

Once you are certain the casualty is unconscious be sure he has a patent airway and can breathe.
Look for chest movement,
listen with your cheek close to his mouth for breath sounds, and
feel expired air on the side of your cheek.
If the casualty is not breathing or has difficulty in breathing the air passages may be obstructed.

Obstruction often occurs because the relaxed tongue falls on to the posterior pharyngeal wall, but it is occasionally due to foreign bodies—food, dentures, weeds, etc. If the patient is breathing but unconscious place him in the recovery position and if necessary support his chin to maintain the airway. In this position the tongue will fall away from the pharyngeal wall and any vomit will dribble out of the corner of the mouth rather than obstruct the airway or, later on, cause aspiration pneumonia.

1

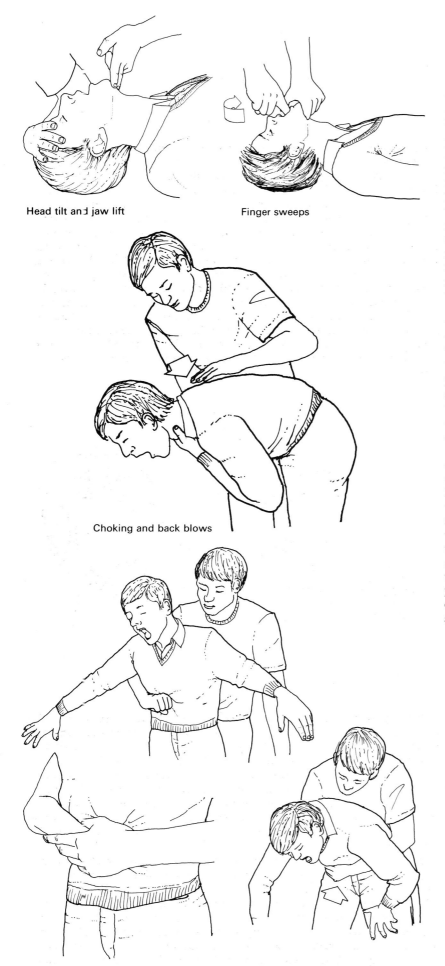

Head tilt and jaw lift

Finger sweeps

Choking and back blows

Heimlich's abdominal thrust

Treatment of obstructed airway—Establishing and maintaining an airway is the single most useful resuscitative manoeuvre the rescuer can perform. The aim is to extend, not hyperextend, the neck (thus lifting the tongue off the posterior wall of the pharynx), and this is best achieved by lifting the chin forwards with the finger and thumb of one hand while pressing the forehead backwards with the heel of the other hand. If this fails to establish an airway see if there is obstruction by a foreign body. Try to remove this first by finger sweeps in the mouth if the jaw is relaxed. If this is not successful try firm blows to the back, which may dislodge a foreign body by compressing what air remains in the lungs and causing an upward force behind the obstructing material.

In the conscious patient the most effective way of removing any obstruction is to gain the victim's confidence and encourage him to cough. This allows the patient to use the muscles in his bronchi together with his chest muscles to produce as much pressure as possible with the air remaining in his lungs. If this fails ask him to lean over a chair and deliver firm blows to the centre of his back, thus calling gravity to your aid as well.

If back blows and finger sweeps fail abdominal thrusts can be tried. Stand behind a conscious patient and put both your arms round him. Make a fist of one hand immediately below the xiphisternum, grasp it with the other hand, and pull both hands firmly and suddenly up towards the patient's upper thoracic spine. If the object is not expelled, repeat the manoeuvre six or seven times. For an unconscious patient the same manoeuvre can be attempted with the patient lying supine and the rescuer astride him or to one side at the level of the pelvis. Alternate abdominal thrusts with back blows.

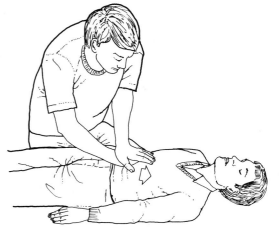

Abdominal thrust in unconscious patient

Breathing

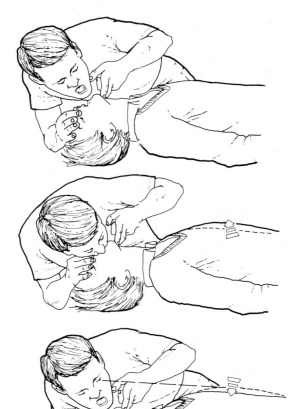

If the patient is not breathing, regardless of the cause, start expired air respiration immediately. Take a deep breath, seal your lips firmly around those of the patient, and (while still maintaining an airway by lifting the jaw with one hand) pinch the nose with the fingers of the other hand (which is already pressing on to the forehead). Breathe out until you see the patient's chest expand and then lift your head away so that the patient can exhale and you can take another breath of air; the chest should rise and fall as you breathe in and out of the patient.

Two complete breaths are sufficient initially, then check the carotid pulse. If it is present then maintain respiration by providing expired air resuscitation at the rate of 12 to 16 breaths a minute. Each breath should expand the victim's chest but not cause overdistension, as this will allow air to enter the oesophagus and stomach. Gastric distension not only causes vomiting (which we are likely to notice and to aspirate), but also passive regurgitation into the lungs, which is not so easily detected. Once the patient starts to breathe for himself, place him in the recovery position.

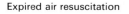

Expired air resuscitation

Circulation

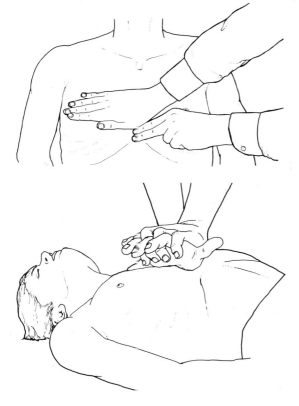

If the patient does not have a pulse in a major artery (preferably the carotid but if the neck is injured the pulse may be felt at the femoral artery) then circulation must be established with chest compressions.

After you have given two initial breaths compress the chest (in an adult) by 1½–2 inches (4–5 cm) at a rate of 80 compressions a minute making sure that the downward compressions occupy more than half of the cycle of compression and relaxation. At a rate of 80 a minute there is time to do 15 compressions and pause to give two inflations so that there will be 60 compressions overall each minute at a rate of 15 compressions to two inflations.

The positioning of your hands and shoulders for this technique is important. Feel along the ribs until you come to the xiphisternum; place two fingers at the base of the xiphisternum, then place the heel of the other hand above these two fingers on the sternum. Put your second hand on top of the first hand and align your shoulders above this position with the arms straight. Press down firmly, not allowing your elbows to flex. Moving from the shoulders, compress down and up counting "one and two and three," etc, until you get to 15, when you pause for the two inflations.

3

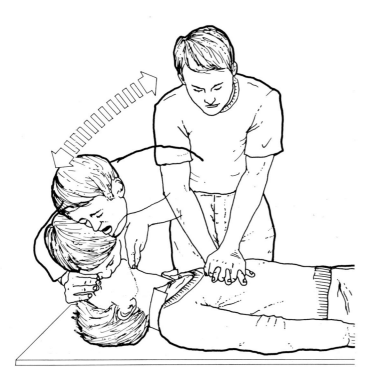

One rescuer cardiopulmonary resuscitation

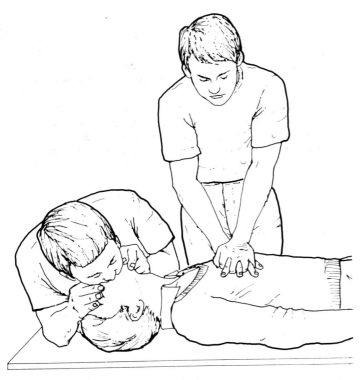

Two rescuer cardiopulmonary resuscitation

When two rescuers are present one is responsible for inflating the lungs and the other for chest compressions. The sequence should start with the first rescuer assessing the patient, establishing an airway, and giving two inflations. He should then pause while the second rescuer compresses the chest. This should still be at a rate of at least 80 compressions a minute, but with a pause after every five compressions to allow the first rescuer (who has been maintaining the airway throughout the chest compressions) to interpose one lung inflation, allowing 1–1½ seconds for this inflation and deflation before the next five compressions are given. This pause can be shorter if the victim is intubated, as faster expiratory flow rates will not distend the stomach. When the chest compressor becomes tired the rescuers exchange positions.

It is difficult to teach basic life support by a textbook or even on patients, but luckily many commercial training aids and manikins are available for training and practice.

Dangers of resuscitation

Until recently the main concern in resuscitation was for the patient, but attention has recently been directed towards the rescuer, particularly in the light of fears about the transmission of the acquired immune deficiency syndrome. No case of AIDS has been transferred by mouth to mouth resuscitation and it does not seem to behave as a saliva borne disease. Research on AIDS is still in its infancy, however, and doctors will be asked about airway adjuncts. Adequate resuscitation can still be performed if a barrier is used between the patient and the doctor (such as a pocket face mask or some form of airway). The main requirement of these devices is that they should not hinder an adequate flow of air and not provide too great a dead space. Resuscitation must not be delayed until such a device is at hand.

1 Safar P. Ventilatory efficacy of mouth to mouth artificial respiration. Airway obstruction during manual and mouth to mouth artificial respiration. *JAMA* 1958; **167**: 335–1.
2 Kouwenhoven WB, Jude JR, Knickerbocker CG. Closed chest cardiac massage. *JAMA* 1960; **173**: 1064–7.
3 Safar P, Brown TC, Holtey WH, *et al.* Ventilation and circulation with closed chest cardiac massage. *JAMA* 1961; **176**: 574–80.
4 Heimlich HJ. A life saving manoeuvre to save food-choking, *JAMA* 1975; **234**: 398–401.
5 American Heart Association. 1985 National Conference on Standards and Guidelines for Cardiopulmonary Resuscitation and Emergency Cardiac Care. Standards and guidelines for cardiopulmonary resuscitation and emergency cardiac care. *JAMA* 1986; **255**: 2843–989.
6 Melker R. Asynchronous and other alternative methods of ventilation during CPR. *Ann Emerg Med* 1984; **13**: 758–61.

VENTRICULAR FIBRILLATION

DOUGLAS CHAMBERLAIN

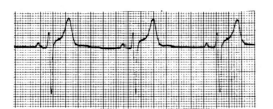

Sinus rhythm

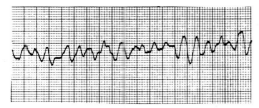

Coarse ventricular fibrillation

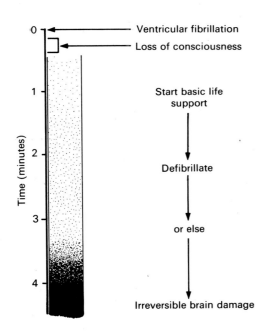

Ventricular fibrillation is electrical anarchy within the ventricular myocardium. The normal heart beat is generated by a sequence of depolarisation, mechanical contraction, and active relaxation of the heart muscle that spreads rapidly throughout the ventricular myocardium in an orderly fashion—exquisitely designed to propel blood rather than simply to expel it.

In ventricular fibrillation coordination of the beat breaks down totally, so that electrical depolarisation and contraction of fibres become apparently random. The muscle continues to work after fibrillation supervenes, but contraction in one group of fibres is counteracted by relaxation in neighbouring fibres. Inspection of the ventricles would show them to be quivering rather than beating. This movement gradually diminishes owing to progressive ischaemia, as no blood flows through the coronary arteries during cardiac arrest. Ventricular fibrillation therefore passes imperceptibly into irreversible and untreatable asystole (but note that asystole occurring as a primary arrhythmia or as an abrupt result of therapy does sometimes respond to treatment). The changes are reflected in the electrocardiogram: the distinctive QRS/T complexes of the coordinated heart beat are replaced by a continuous random wave form, which usually starts as a coarse pattern and becomes progressively finer as the quivering of the myocardium ceases.

Ventricular fibrillation is the most common mechanism of cardiac arrest in patients with ischaemic heart disease (the others are asystole and electromechanical dissociation, considered in the next chapter). Ventricular fibrillation occurs as a complication of myocardial infarction, within the first few hours in uncomplicated cases but less predictably and often later in patients with heart failure or cardiogenic shock. It may also occur unheralded, in the absence of pain or other symptoms, and thus cause sudden cardiac death. The old assumption that a new myocardial infarction is an invariable prelude to sudden cardiac death is incorrect, but most victims do have severe underlying obstructive coronary disease with some recent instability (such as rupture of an atheromatous plaque) that caused localised ischaemia as a trigger for the arrhythmia. Whatever the precipitating cause, consciousness is lost within 10 to 20 seconds of the onset of ventricular fibrillation.

Appropriate first aid (basic life support) or defibrillation, or both, must be provided within two to four minutes if cerebral damage is not to be irreversible. It also becomes more difficult to restore the heart beat if resuscitation is delayed.

Electrical defibrillation

Ventricular fibrillation may rarely remit spontaneously or as a result of a precordial thump; but these possibilities exist only very briefly after the onset of the arrhythmia, presumably because the loss of coronary flow exacerbates the electrical instability. No conclusive evidence exists that any drug can abolish ventricular fibrillation in

5

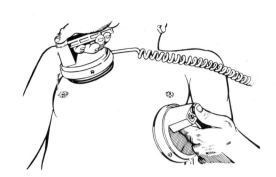

Paddle positions for manual defibrillator

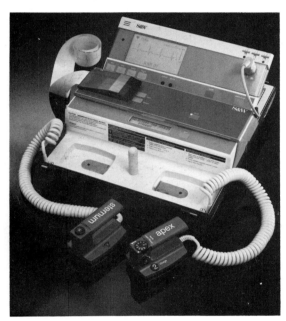

Manual defibrillator

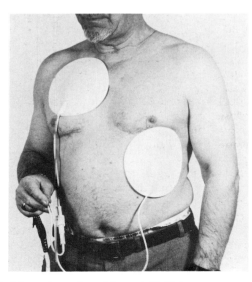

Paddle positions for advisory defibrillator

man even if the circulation is maintained by basic life support. The only effective treatment for established ventricular fibrillation is electrical defibrillation, and the quicker this can be provided the better the prospects for long term success.

Defibrillation is a simple treatment. A large electrical impulse ("shock") is delivered to the heart through the chest wall. This causes depolarisation of all the myocardial cells not at that moment totally refractory. If enough cells are depolarised then the incessant fibrillatory wave forms of random depolarisation are no longer propagated throughout the ventricular myocardium, and after a brief interval the normal impulses transmitted through the conducting pathways of the heart take over control of the heart beat. Effective mechanical activity usually begins at once, but may be delayed for a few moments or even longer after restoration of a satisfactory electrocardiogram.

Defibrillators are usually powered by a rechargeable battery but some are mains operated. Few controls are necessary. Apart from an on-off switch, the equipment allows for variation in the energy stored in the capacitor for discharge through the chest wall. Calibration points for delivered energy, including 200 and 360 J, are usual (older models show calibration in stored energy, 100 J stored being equivalent to 80 J delivered). The shock is delivered by well protected hand held electrodes, or paddles. They have an integral discharge button so that the operator can control the timing of the delivery of the shock.

Means must be available to dump any unused charge. Most portable defibrillators have a monitoring facility with an oscilloscope to show heart rhythm; the defibrillation paddles act also as electrodes for transmitting the electrocardiogram.

For defibrillation, one electrode should be placed below the right clavicle and the other over the points designated as V4 and V5 for the electrocardiogram—that is, a little outside the position of the normal apex beat. The polarity of the plates is unimportant so their position is interchangeable. Impedance at the interface of plate and skin must be kept to a minimum. Electrode jelly can be used for this purpose, but it tends to spread during chest compression with the risk that subsequent shocks will arc across the chest surface. Conducting gel pads should be used instead and removed between shocks. The pressure of plate against pad and skin also determines impedance and should therefore be firm. The operator must ensure that neither he nor anyone else is touching the patient when the shock is delivered.

The procedures are simpler when automatic or semiautomatic defibrillators are used. In these circumstances the operator usually has only modest training in advanced life support, and drug treatment may well be irrelevant. The sequence to be followed for defibrillation depends on the instrument that is used, but all that are now available have simplicity as a keynote. In general, the operator follows instructions that appear on a display panel that is usually of the liquid crystal variety. With the adhesive pads correctly attached to the patient and the machine turned on, the first instruction is to wait while the heart rhythm is automatically tested against the algorithms within the machine. Basic life support must be interrupted while the rhythm is being analysed. The delay may seem unacceptably long to rescuers who understand the need for maintaining the circulation, but studies have shown that the delay overall tends to be less than with manual machines (even when they are used by skilled operators). A fully automatic defibrillator should eventually signal that a shock is to be given (with advice to stand clear) or that no shock is advised. The shock at a preset energy level (usually 200 J) follows without further intervention. In the case of the more common semiautomatic ("advisory") defibrillators, the operator is advised to press a button that releases the discharge if a shock is indicated. Some human control is therefore retained. This permits a final check that defibrillation is appropriate, but carries with it the onus of decision making that can be disadvantageous. On balance, however, semiautomatic defibrillators are considered preferable in most circumstances. The possibility exists for repeat shocks, though often with a preset limit. Some equipment permits an increase in the strength of the discharge for refractory arrhythmias.

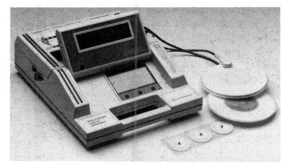

Advisory or semiautomatic defibrillator

The implications of the development of automatic and semiautomatic defibrillators have not been widely appreciated. There is no longer any justification for a front line ambulance to be without a defibrillator and staff capable of using it. First aid workers responsible for large crowds, health care professionals working with patients judged to be at high risk of fibrillation, and the rescue services should also be equipped and trained. The training takes a maximum of four hours, and the cost of the equipment is modest in relation to its potential value.

Guidelines for defibrillation procedures that were laid down by the Resuscitation Council of the United Kingdom have recently been revised. The sequence of energies and the details of drug administration given here are based on these new recommendations.

Procedure

```
1   Basic life support
2   Give shock: 200 J
3   Check major pulse within 3s
4   If no pulse give 15 chest compressions
5   Place paddles and read ECG
6   Use shock sequence as below
```

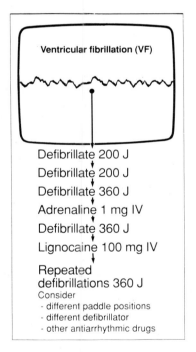

Ventricular fibrillation (VF)

Defibrillate 200 J
↓
Defibrillate 200 J
↓
Defibrillate 360 J
↓
Adrenaline 1 mg IV
↓
Defibrillate 360 J
↓
Lignocaine 100 mg IV
↓
Repeated
defibrillations 360 J
Consider
- different paddle positions
- different defibrillator
- other antiarrhythmic drugs

If the cardiac arrest is witnessed or monitored, the first intervention should be a precordial thump with the ulnar margin of the closed fist. This is delivered from about 20 cm above the chest sharply on the junction between the lower and middle thirds of the sternum. Though of most value in asystole or ventricular tachycardia, a thump can also be effective on rare occasions within a few seconds of the onset of ventricular fibrillation. It carries little risk and takes only a few moments.

If the thump is unsuccessful and a defibrillator is immediately available, defibrillation should be attempted at once. In most cases, however, definitive electrical treatment cannot be administered for a minute or more even within an intensive care area; the victim should then receive basic life support as an important interim measure. Basic life support should not be interrupted for intubation or placing intravenous lines if a shock—which has the top priority—can be delivered quickly. If possible, one rescuer should continue chest compression while a second charges the defibrillator to 200 J so that interruption of basic life support is minimised before delivery of this and subsequent shocks.

A monitoring oscilloscope may take five to 10 seconds to "recover" after delivery of the shock so no interpretation of the electrocardiogram is possible during this period; the procedure after defibrillation should ensure that no time is wasted without circulatory support while the rescuer gazes at an inoperative screen. The following routine is suggested:

(1) give shock,
(2) check major pulse within three seconds,
(3) if no pulse administer 15 more chest compressions,
(4) only then attempt to read electrocardiogram.

If coordinated rhythm has returned chest compression is unlikely to precipitate recurrence of fibrillation and it has no serious effect on the beating heart. If fibrillation is still present further shocks are given at 200 J and 360 J using the procedures outlined above. Basic life support is continued at all times except when the shocks are delivered.

Failure of these initial attempts at rapid defibrillation may be due to hypoxia or acidosis: the ideal treatment for both is hyperventilation after intubation, though outside hospital this will not always be practicable. (Ventilation is more effective than sodium bicarbonate for reversing acidosis at this stage: without efficient elimination of carbon dioxide, sodium bicarbonate may even worsen intracellular acidosis).

Constant electrocardiographic monitoring will be needed in any prolonged cardiac arrest, and adhesive electrodes should be used for the subsequent phase of the resuscitation attempt.

Continue CPR for up to 2 min. after each drug. Do not interrupt CPR for more than 10 sec., except for defibrillation. If an I.V. line cannot be established, consider giving double doses of adrenaline or lignocaine via an endotracheal tube.

PROLONGED RESUSCITATION:
Give 1 mg adrenaline IV every 5 minutes.
Consider 50 mmol sodium bicarbonate
(50 ml. of 8.4%) or according to blood gas results.

POST RESUSCITATION CARE
Check
- arterial blood gases
- electrolytes
- chest x-ray
Observe monitor and treat patient
in an intensive care area.

Drug administration is recommended if the first three shocks are unsuccessful; a venous cannula should therefore be inserted with the tip placed as centrally as possible using a route that is best suited to the experience of the operator. The order should be as follows: adrenaline 1 mg (10 ml of 1 in 10 000 solution) before the fourth shock and lignocaine 100 mg before the fifth shock. Routines for checking the pulse should be repeated as described above. Before further defibrillating attempts are made, basic life support should be continued for up to two minutes after each drug has been administered to allow the possibility of the agents reaching the heart. A "chaser" infusion of 5% dextrose may help, though any drug effects will at best be very slow in onset. If an intravenous line cannot be established, the endotracheal route may be used for the adrenaline and lignocaine, but this method of administration is associated with variable absorption and is not recommended as first choice. Double doses of the drugs are used to compensate for the poorer availability, but the formula is at best empirical. Note that sodium bicarbonate, which has appreciable disadvantages during resuscitation, is not used at this stage, which now entails only two drugs and not three as previously.

Patients who remain in ventricular fibrillation have no chance of recovery, so further efforts at defibrillation may be justified when drug treatment seems to have failed. Consider a different paddle position: the original orientation may have given an unsuspected high impedance pathway. Front to back on the left chest should achieve greatest current density at the heart, though this may be difficult to achieve safely in a heavy patient. Axilla to axilla is an alternative, though unproved. The use of a different defibrillator for refractory cases is also wise, even if no fault is suspected in the original instrument. Sometimes slightly higher energies can be delivered if paddle pressure is increased, and ECG electrode jelly does offer a lower impedance than the defibrillation pads that are preferable for routine use. (Jelly that has been used early in a resuscitation attempt can spread over the chest and cause ineffective arcing of later shocks.)

For truly refractory ventricular fibrillation the use of bretylium tosylate should be considered. Experimental evidence suggests that this has better antifibrillatory properties than other antiarrhythmic drugs. A dose of 400 mg (usually 4 ampoules in the United Kingdom) should be given by intravenous injection. Bretylium achieves its effect relatively slowly, so once this drug is used the rescuers should be prepared to continue chest compression and defibrillation attempts for a further 20-30 minutes. This will be appropriate only in a few cases.

Sodium bicarbonate does have a role in very prolonged resuscitations, provided that ventilation is fully effective. The initial dose is 50 mmol (50 ml of 8·4%) intravenously, and this can be repeated if indicated by blood gas results. Adrenaline may also be given again if early attempts at resuscitation are unsuccessful, principally with the objective of maintaining the efficiency of basic life support. Experimentally it can favour blood flow to the brain, which otherwise tends to be compromised by collapse of the extrathoracic great vessels. The usual dose of 1 mg can be repeated at up to five minute intervals.

No recommendation has been made for the maximum number of shocks that should be administered, because circumstances vary between patients. If the prospects for resuscitation had seemed to be good and if striving is fully appropriate, then an end point may not be reached for about an hour. By that time, the fibrillatory waveform may be so fine as to be indistinguishable from asystole. There can be little prospect of success at this stage. This ominous development must be distinguished from the brief period of true asystole that is common after successful defibrillation. This is treated initially only by continued basic life support, and drug treatment for systole should not be considered for at least a minute or two lest fresh fibrillation is induced unnecessarily

If fibrillation does recur for any reason and at any time, the whole sequence outlined above should be started from the beginning. Thus the first shock would again be 200 J.

Summary

(1) The hopeful phase: three shocks at 200 J, 200 J, 360 J.

(2) The struggling phase: two shocks at 360 J after adrenaline and lignocaine. Patient intubated if possible.

(3) The desperate phase: three or more shocks at 360 J with different electrode position or different defibrillator.

Though improvements will doubtless be made as skill in resuscitation increases, the guidelines can ensure that relatively few treated patients die in ventricular fibrillation and only those with irreversible myocardial damage are likely to be converted to intractable asystole.

ASYSTOLE AND ELECTROMECHANICAL DISSOCIATION

A JOHN CAMM

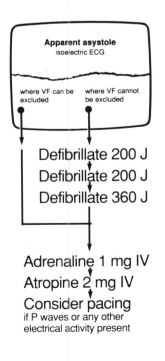

The three main mechanisms of cardiac arrest are ventricular fibrillation, ventricular asystole, and electromechanical dissociation. About 25% of arrests in hospital and 10% of those outside hospital are asystolic. Less than 3% of sudden cardiac arrests that occur outside hospital, but a very much higher percentage (30–70%) of arrests occurring in hospital, are due to electromechanical dissociation. Both asystole and electromechanical dissociation have a much worse prognosis than ventricular fibrillation.

Asystole

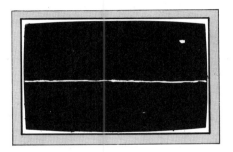

Onset of asystole

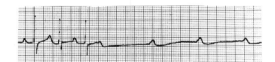

Apparent asystole
isoelectric ECG

where VF can be excluded   where VF cannot be excluded

Defibrillate 200 J
Defibrillate 200 J
Defibrillate 360 J

Adrenaline 1 mg IV
Atropine 2 mg IV
Consider pacing
if P waves or any other electrical activity present

Asystole is a form of cardiac arrest characterised by ventricular standstill due to the suppression of natural or artificial pacemakers. Myocardial disease, electrolyte aberration, anoxia, or drugs acting on the myocardium may suppress idioventricular rhythms responsible for maintaining cardiac output when either higher or artificial pacemakers fail or when atrioventricular conduction is interrupted. Strong cholinergic activity may suddenly depress the function of the sinus or atrioventricular nodes, especially when sympathetic stimulation is reduced—for example, by ischaemia, infarction, or β blockade.

Asystole is diagnosed when no ventricular activity is seen on the electrocardiogram, but a mistaken diagnosis may be made if the electrical recording system is faulty or wrongly connected. The leads, connections, gain, and brilliance of the monitor must be checked. Ventricular fibrillation may be mistaken for asystole, especially if only one lead is monitored or if the fibrillatory activity is of low voltage. Asystole may also give way to ventricular fibrillation caused by anoxia, acidaemia, and hyperkalaemia provoked by the asystole.

Management – Fine ventricular fibrillation may simulate the electrocardiographic appearance of asystole (flat trace). When ventricular fibrillation is suspected the conventional series of capacitor charges (200 J, 200 J, and 360 J) should be delivered (see previous chapter).

The administration of vasopressor drugs such as adrenaline is crucial to adequate cerebral and coronary perfusion during cardiopulmonary resuscitation. α Adrenergic stimulation produces intense vasoconstriction in other vascular beds and prevents coronary and cerebral arterial collapse during chest compression. In addition, the β adrenergic effect of adrenaline increases the rate of discharge of the nodes and the working idioventricular myocardium.

Theoretically atropine should relieve cholinergic depression of function of the sinus and atrioventricular nodes, and there is ample animal and clinical evidence of this during the autonomic chaos after myocardial infarction. This does not necessarily translate into improved survival from asystolic arrest, and in animals atropine does not seem to improve the outcome from cardiac arrest. A retrospective analysis of 43 asystolic patients given atropine, however, showed successful resuscitation in six (compared with none of 41 controls).

9

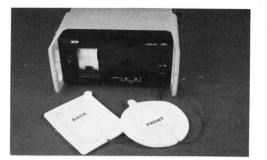

Cardiac pacing is undoubtedly effective when applied to the immediate resuscitation of patients with asystole due to sudden and predominant failure of sinus node discharge or to atrioventricular block. Pacing is not as successful, however, when asystolic arrest occurs because of extensive myocardial or systemic derangement. Generally dismal results have been reported; for example, in 50 asystolic prehospital cardiac arrests managed with transcutaneous pacing, ventricular capture was achieved in 26 and a pulse obtained in only five. The traumatic hazards of transcutaneous pacing (through a needle inserted directly into the myocardium) may be avoided by transthoracic pacing (from electrodes applied to the skin of the thorax). Although transthoracic pacing has proved successful, though often uncomfortable, for elective pacing, it is disappointing for the emergency pacing of victims of asystolic cardiac arrest. Pacing the ventricles via the oesophagus is awkward and almost always unsuccessful. Transvenous ventricular pacing should be considered if there is evidence of P wave activity with no ventricular complexes or if very slow rhythms are present.

Retrospective studies and a prospective study have shown that calcium is not useful for managing asystolic cardiac arrest.

The profound hypoxia of severe asthma may give rise to asystole. Patients must be intubated and ventilated with 100% oxygen immediately. Vigorous resuscitation attempts are always indicated and may sometimes be successful.

Electromechanical dissociation

Electromechanical dissociation is profound myocardial pump failure despite normal or near normal electrical excitation. It is rare outside hospital and more common in hospital patients. It usually occurs secondary to drugs or mechanical embarrassment such as cardiac tamponade, pulmonary embolism, tension pneumothorax, intracardiac thrombus or tumour, or myocardial rupture or exsanguination. Primary electromechanical dissociation is diagnosed after mechanical causes and hypovolaemia have been excluded and is a failure of excitation-contraction coupling seen most often in the setting of acute inferior wall myocardial infarction. Its mechanism is not understood, but intracellular acidosis and autonomic effects are suspected. It may occur as the end point of prolonged ventricular fibrillation and may be produced experimentally by anoxia, acidosis, or perfusion with a calcium free medium.

Electromechanical dissociation in a patient with acute myocardial infarction. Despite an apparently near normal cardiac rhythm there was no blood pressure.

Causes of electromechanical dissociation

1 *Primary electromechanical dissociation (failure of excitation-contraction coupling)*

   Myocardial infarction (particularly inferior wall)
   Drugs (β blockers and calcium antagonists) or toxins
   Electrolyte abnormalities (such as hypocalcaemia, hyperkalaemia)
   Atrial thrombus or tumour (myxoma)

2 *Secondary electromechanical dissociation (mechanical embarrassment to cardiac output)*

   Pericardial tamponade
   Cardiac rupture
   Pulmonary embolism
   Tension pneumothorax
   Hypovolaemia
   Prosthetic heart valve occlusion

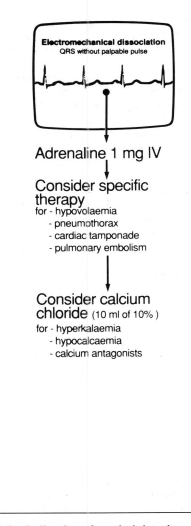

Electromechanical dissociation
QRS without palpable pulse

Adrenaline 1 mg IV

Consider specific therapy
for - hypovolaemia
 - pneumothorax
 - cardiac tamponade
 - pulmonary embolism

Consider calcium chloride (10 ml of 10%)
for - hyperkalaemia
 - hypocalcaemia
 - calcium antagonists

Definite indications for administering calcium in cardiac arrest

1 Known or suspected hypocalcaemia
2 Recent massive transfusion
3 Known or suspected hyperkalaemia
4 Calcium antagonist toxicity
5 "Last resort" in electromechanical dissociation or asystole, especially if wide QRS

Management—Exclude or treat any mechanical cause. For example, hypovolaemia, cardiac tamponade, tension pneumothorax, pulmonary embolism, and other mechanical embarrassments to effective cardiac action may present with a dangerously low cardiac output and a normal or near normal QRS complex on the electrocardiogram. These physical causes of electromechanical dissociation must be treated by appropriate means, such as volume expansion for hypovolaemia or pericardial tap for a rapidly accumulating pericardial effusion. If primary electromechanical dissociation is present pressor agents such as adrenaline or methoxamine (both α_1 agonists) are an essential adjunct to cardiopulmonary resuscitation. Theoretically the inotropic effect of β 'stimulation (adrenaline or isoprenaline) should be advantageous but this has not been confirmed.

In electromechanical dissociation calcium may be effective, especially when the QRS complex is wide (0·12 s or more). Several large retrospective studies have suggested that intravenous administration of calcium was not associated with an increased survival, but in the only prospective randomised study of patients with electromechanical dissociation, eight of 48 who received 5 ml calcium chloride 10% were resuscitated compared with only two of 42 who received saline. Success with calcium infusion was limited to those with QRS complex widening or electrocardiographic evidence of acute ischaemia (T wave and ST segment abnormalities).

The case for calcium administration is not proved, but its use is reasonable if no other treatment is effective. Calcium infusion is specifically indicated when hypocalcaemia, hyperkalaemia, or calcium antagonist toxicity is present. It must be remembered, however, that hypercalcaemia and calcium overload sufficient to cause cardiac or cerebral cell death may complicate the intravenous use of calcium during a cardiac arrest. There is some experimental evidence that calcium antagonists may preserve cerebral blood flow and function during cardiac arrest and may be particularly useful in resuscitating patients who have suffered an arrest because of electromechanical dissociation, but there is practically no clinical experience of this.

Cardiac pacing is not usually successful, although restoring atrioventricular synchrony with dual chamber pacing or the use of paired and coupled ventricular pacing may occasionally be helpful.

Conclusions

Resuscitation from cardiac asystole or from electromechanical dissociation is considerably less satisfactory than resuscitation from ventricular fibrillation. Nevertheless, considerable recent progress has challenged old dogma and introduced new and potentially rewarding treatments.

THE AIRWAY AT RISK

ROBERT S SIMONS, T HILARY HOWELLS

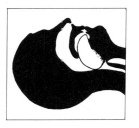
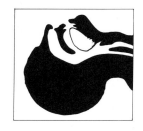

Failure to maintain a patent airway is a common cause of avoidable death in unconscious patients. The principles of airway management after cardiac arrest are the same as those used during anaesthesia or resuscitation after major trauma. Patency of the airway may be impaired by loss of normal muscle tone or by obstruction, including contamination by foreign material from the mouth, nasopharynx, oesophagus, or stomach.

Airway patency

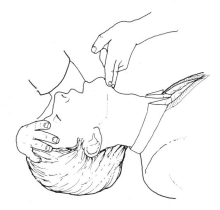

Head tilt and jaw lift

In the unconscious patient relaxation of the tongue, neck, and pharyngeal muscles causes soft tissue obstruction of the supraglottic airway. Correction using long established manoeuvres includes head tilt and jaw lift or jaw thrust. The use of neck lift is no longer recommended in first aid manuals because it leaves one hand committed behind the patient's neck and it may be dangerous if there is an unstable injury of the cervical spine. Head tilt will relieve obstruction in 80% of patients, and chin lift or jaw thrust will further improve overall patency but tend to oppose the lips. In some of these patients airway obstruction may persist, particularly during expiration, probably because of nasal airway obstruction caused by a "flap valve" effect of soft palate and nasopharyngeal tissues, as in snoring.

Safar's triple manoeuvre requires the rescuer to open the patient's mouth while performing head tilt and jaw thrust.[1] It is difficult to maintain, especially when performing artificial respiration at the same time.

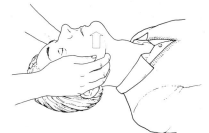

Jaw thrust

Recovery posture

Patients with adequate spontaneous ventilation and circulation, but who cannot safeguard their own airway, will be at risk in the supine position. Turning the patient laterally into the "coma" or "recovery" position allows the tongue to fall forward, with less risk of pharyngeal obstruction, and fluid in the mouth can drain out instead of soiling the trachea and lungs.

Recovery positions range from a true lateral posture (with either upper or lower leg flexed) to the semiprone, depending on the relative tilt of the pelvis and shoulders and attitude of the arms. Several authorities favour the lower arm extended behind the back to prevent reverse roll. The semiprone posture has been preferred as producing better airway patency and drainage and greater stability during transport, but the casualty's face, colour, and chest movement are more difficult to observe in this position, and ventilation may be impaired. Moreover, the patient is inconveniently positioned if he has to be turned supine again for further resuscitation.

The patient may lie on either side. Some argue that emergency tracheal intubation may be performed more easily with the patient lying on his left rather than right side, but a full stomach is more liable to compression and regurgitation in this position. Some first aid texts recommend that unconscious patients with associated chest injuries are best positioned with the uninjured lung uppermost. The pathophysiology of thoracic injury is such that there may be some circumstances when this may not be appropriate.

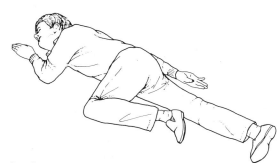

Semiprone recovery position

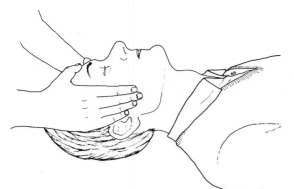

In line cervical stabilisation

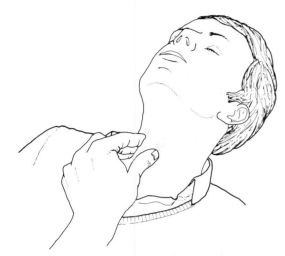

Sellick's manoeuvre of cricoid pressure

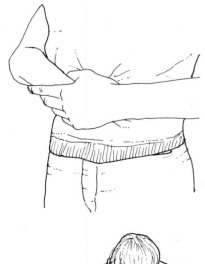

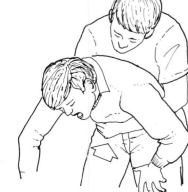

Heimlich's abdominal thrust

Spinal injury

Casualties with suspected spinal injuries need careful handling and should be managed in the supine aligned position with constant attention to the airway. If the recovery posture has to be adopted the patient should be "logrolled" into a true lateral position by several rescuers in unison to avoid spinal rotation. The semiprone position is not suitable in these circumstances because considerable rotation of the neck is required to prevent the subject lying on his face. If the head or upper chest is injured, bony neck injury should be assumed until excluded by lateral cervical spine radiography. Immobilisation in a neutral position using traction, a rigid collar, or sandbags is imperative. The neck must not be actively flexed or extended, and nasal airways and intubation may be preferrable to oral techniques.

Vomiting and regurgitation

Rescuers should always be aware of the risk of contamination of the unprotected airway by fluid or solid debris and should attempt to forestall it. Vomiting and regurgitation are subtly different.

Vomiting happens more commonly during light levels of unconsciousness and may occur as the level of consciousness improves during successful resuscitation. It is an active process of stomach contraction and retrograde propulsion up the oesophagus. Prodromal retching may allow time to put the patient in the lateral recovery position or head down (Trendelenburg) tilt and prepare for suction or manual removal of debris from the mouth and pharynx.

Regurgitation is a passive and often silent flow of stomach contents (typically fluid) up the oesophagus, with the risk of unprotected inhalation and soiling of the lungs. Acidic gastric fluid may cause severe chemical pneumonitis. Failure to maintain a clear airway during spontaneous respiration may also encourage regurgitation because the excessive negative intrathoracic pressure developed during obstructed inspiration may aspirate gastric contents across a weak mucosal flap valve from the stomach to the oesophagus. Recent food or fluid ingestion, obesity, hiatus hernia, intestinal obstruction, and late pregnancy all make regurgitation more probable during resuscitation. Cardiac compression and the use of abdominal binders or counterpulsation also add to the risk of regurgitation.

Gaseous distension of the stomach increases the likelihood of regurgitation and restricts lung expansion. Inadvertent gastric inflation may occur during artificial respiration when rapid lung ventilation is used giving large tidal volumes and high inflation pressures. This is particularly likely when gas powered resuscitators are used with facemasks. These resuscitators should only be used when the patient has been intubated.

The cricoid pressure manoeuvre, recommended by Sellick in 1961,[2] is well known to anaesthetists. Compressing the oesophagus between the cricoid ring and the sixth cervical vertebra prevents passive regurgitation, but it should not be applied during active vomiting. It also serves a useful purpose during resuscitation in preventing undesired gastric inflation, but requires the help of another rescuer.

Choking

Asphyxia caused by the impaction of food or a foreign body in the upper airway is a dramatic and frightening event, which may closely resemble a heart attack. Urgent action is required to avert a catastrophe.[3] In the conscious patient back blows and abdominal thrusts[4] have been widely recommended. Attempts may be made to provoke coughing or vomiting. If these are not successful the patient will become unconscious and collapse. The supine casualty may be given further abdominal thrusts and manual attempts at pharyngeal disimpaction should be undertaken. Visual inspection of the throat with a laryngoscope and the use of Magill forceps or suction is desirable, but such equipment is seldom available at the time of need.

If resuscitation so far has been unsuccessful the ultimate hypoxic arrest may be indistinguishable from other causes of cardiac arrest, and treatment should follow the ABC (airway, breathing, and circulation) routine, although ventilation may be difficult or impossible to perform. On the other hand, the act of forceful chest compression may clear the offending object from the laryngopharynx.

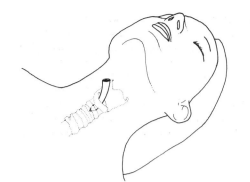

Cricothyrotomy (laryngotomy)

Surgical intervention

If the airway above the vocal cords remains obstructed, for example by a foreign body, faciomaxillary trauma, extrinsic pressure, or inflammation, the manoeuvre of cricothyrotomy (laryngotomy) may be life saving and should not be unduly delayed. Any strong knife, scissor point, large bore cannula, or similar instrument can be used to create an opening through the cricothyroid membrane, although purpose designed cricothyrotomy devices are best if available. Once created an opening of 5–7 mm diameter needs to be maintained. Artificial ventilation may be applied directly to this orifice or tube insert.

Jet ventilation with oxygen at 40–50 psi (3 bar) applied to a 12–14 G cannula cricothyrotomy, can be used as an emergency measure for up to 45 minutes pending a surgical cricothyrotomy or tracheostomy. To allow adequate time for expiration, a cycle of inflation for one second and exhalation for four seconds should be maintained when using this technique. Tracheostomy is technically difficult and should only be undertaken by those trained appropriately.

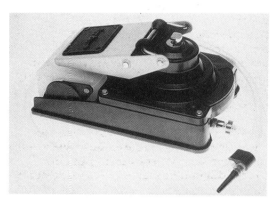

Foot operated suction pump (Ambu)

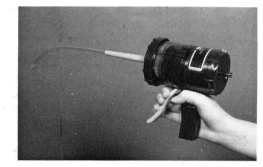

Hand operated suction pump (Vitalograph)

Suction

Equipment for suction clearance of the oropharynx and airways is essential for comprehensive life support. When reviewing the many devices available, considerations of cost, portability, and power supply are paramount. Devices powered by electricity or compressed gas are susceptible to exhaustion of the power supply at a critical time, and battery operated devices need regular recharging or battery replacement. Hand or foot operated pumps are particularly suitable for field use and for the occasional user. Ease of cleaning and simple reassembly are important factors. The use of rigid wide bore plastic or metal suction cannulae can be supplemented by soft plastic suction catheters when necessary. A "suction booster", which traps fluid debris in a reservoir close to the patient, may improve suction capability.

Expired air resuscitation

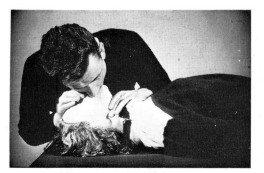

Mouth to mouth resuscitation

If, despite adequate clearance of the patient's airway, spontaneous respiration is absent, artificial ventilation must be started. Earlier manual methods have been superceded universally by intermittent positive pressure techniques, which produce better ventilation. Expired air ventilation exploits the rescuer's expired air to achieve good lung expansion. Although expired air is less rich in oxygen than ambient air (16% v 21%), the resulting oxygenation is acceptable.

The mouth to mouth technique is widely acclaimed and successfully applied by relatively unskilled rescuers. Nevertheless, during its performance it is difficult for the rescuer concurrently to maintain airway patency, effect an airtight seal with his lips, pinch the nose, and also deliver an adequate ventilatory volume.

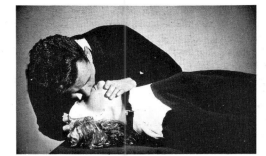

Mouth to nose resuscitation

The alternative route of mouth to nose ventilation was, until recently, popular only with water lifesavers. This method permits maximum head extension and jaw thrust while usefully effecting lip closure. It may be the only option for small mouthed rescuers. Contact with vomit and saliva is reduced, which may make mouth to nose ventilation more acceptable and lessen the risk of infection. Natural nasal resistance limits high inspiratory flow, which might otherwise lead to gastric inflation. If nasopharyngeal obstruction is noted during expiration the rescuer will need to open the casualty's mouth to permit exhalation.

Airway support and ventilation devices

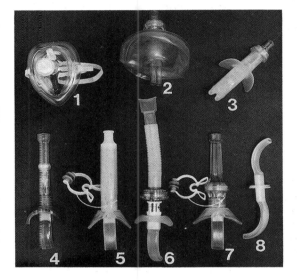

Device	Manufacturer/supplier	Cost
1 Laerdal pocket mask and valve	Laerdal Medical Ltd Goodmead Road Orpington, Kent BR6 0HX	£ 6.00
2 SealEasy/ VentEasy mask-airway	Respironics Monroeville PA 15146, USA	£10.00
3 Dual-Aid	Vitalograph Ltd Maids Moreton Buckingham MK18 1SW	£ 6.75
4 Brook airway (professional model)	G H Wood Ltd 251–5 Moseley Road Birmingham B12 0EN	£12.42
5 Hilt-way	Medifield Ltd Hares Farm, Surlingham Norwich NR14 7DJ	£13.50
6 Sussex valve airway	Tandisdale Medical Ltd Forest Row, E Sussex RH18 5AA	£12.00
7 Lifeway (Weinmann)	Albert Waeschle Ltd 123–5 Old Christchurch Road Bournemouth BH1 1EX	£15.00
8 Safar S airway	Portex Ltd Hythe, Kent CT21 6JL	£ 4.26

Shield devices, comprising a plastic sheet with incorporated filter or protection valve, are also available (at about £1–£2) from the following manufacturers: Bioglan Laboratories Ltd, Wilbury Way, Hitchin SG4 0TW (Bioglan Microshield); Johnson & Johnson, Slough, Berks SL1 1XR (Life Aid); Laerdal Medical (Resusci Face Shield); Portex (Resusciade); and Rorer Pharmaceuticals, Eastbourne (Microshield).

Resuscitation airways are devices that may be used to maintain airway patency, improve spontaneous breathing, or provide a mouthpiece for artificial ventilation if required. Some afford protection to the rescuer and some isolate the airway against pulmonary soiling from gastric aspiration.

Mouth to mouth resuscitation can be physically unpleasant for the rescuer, and there has been public concern about the risk of infection. This has led to an increasing demand for small and inexpensive airway adjuncts that will protect against direct patient contact and communicable diseases.

An extension of the concept of a handkerchief moulded over the patient's face are devices that comprise a plastic sheet incorporating a central bite block with a filter or one way patient valve. They are compact and inexpensive, but are difficult to seal effectively and some tend to have high resistance.

Tongue support

The classic Guedel airway used in anaesthesia improves patency but often requires supplementary jaw support. In lightly comatose patients it may cause oropharyngeal stimulation and vomiting. Soft nasopharyngeal tubes are less stimulating but may cause nasopharyngeal bleeding, and they require some skill for insertion. These simple airways are also suitable for use with mask ventilation.

The reversible Safar S shaped double airway consists of a medium and a large Guedel airway placed back to back. The uninserted airway provides a port for expired air ventilation, if required, and provides some protection for the rescuer.

The Brook airway provides a ventilation port and rescuer protection using a non-return valve. The air flow resistance for rescuer and victim alike is high, and the valve may be lost if the unit is dismantled. The all purpose model is easy to insert but offers no effective tongue support. The professional model has a longer (7 cm) airway, which provides limited tongue support.

More recently new ventilation devices have become available with improved valves for rescuer protection, for example, the Hilt-way, Lifeway, SealEasy/VentEasy, and Sussex airways. The Dual-Aid has the advantage of optional use through the nose or mouth.

Ventilation masks

Ventilation masks offer protection to the rescuer against direct contact with patients, especially if used in conjunction with a non-rebreathing valve. The rescuer blows through a mask firmly applied to the casualty's face. Examples include the Laerdal pocket mask and MTM resuscitator. During expired air resuscitation the rescuer uses two hands to maintain an airtight seal with the mask on the face while also lifting the jaw. It should be remembered, however, that air flow normally takes place through the nose during mask ventilation. Unless oral or nasal airway support devices are used, obstructed expiration may occur and be unrecognised in some patients.

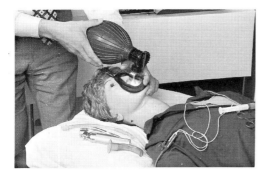

Bag valve mask ventilation

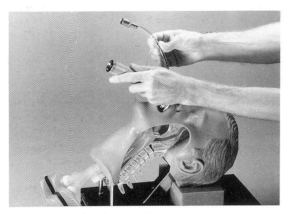

Endotracheal intubation (Ambu)

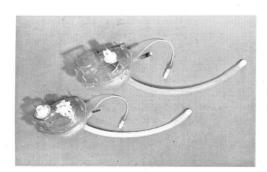

Oesophageal obturators

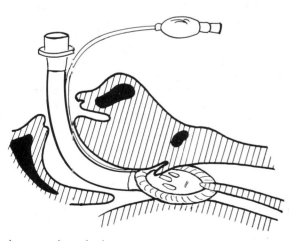

Laryngeal mask airway

Brain laryngeal mask airways are available from Colgate Medical Ltd, Fairacres Estate, Dedworth Road, Windsor, Berks SL4 4LE.

A self refilling bag can be attached to the mask to deliver ambient air, and this can be enriched with oxygen if a source of compressed oxygen is available. The technique requires additional training because it is difficult to apply the mask and lift the jaw with one hand while squeezing the bag with the other.

Several authors have reviewed airway adjuncts, and some have shown that effective ventilatory volumes can be achieved more easily by mouth to mask than by either mouth to mouth or bag valve mask ventilation.[5-9]

Airway isolation

The ultimate in airway management of deeply unconscious patients is tracheal intubation, which requires experience and specific equipment. Traditionally the forté of anaesthetists, this skill has been learnt by emergency medical staff, specialist nurses, and some ambulance staff. The technique essentially entails flexing the subject's neck, extending his head, exposing the epiglottis with a laryngoscope, raising the jaw and base of the tongue forward to expose the larynx, and inserting a curved tube into the trachea. Inflation of the tracheal cuff isolates the airway and permits safe ventilation to be performed. The risks are those of stimulating vomiting in the semiconscious patient, trauma to mouth and larynx, unilateral bronchial intubation, and unrecognised intubation of the oesophagus.

If attempts at tracheal intubation are unsuccessful they must be abandoned without delay and alternative methods of airway control chosen. Techniques for tracheal intubation have been advocated that avoid formal laryngoscopy, but these have limited success even in experienced hands. They include blind nasal intubation, digital manipulation of the tube in the laryngopharynx, or transillumination using lighted tube stylets.

Oesophageal obturators

Oesophageal obturators are popular in the USA. The obturator is a long cuffed tube attached to a face mask. The tube is passed blindly into the oesophagus, and the cuff is then inflated to isolate the oesophagus and stomach from the airway. In the original version the oesophageal obturator tube was blocked distally, and a series of holes at the laryngeal level permitted air blown down the tube to pass from the tube into the larynx. In a later version the oesophageal tube is not terminally sealed, and this allows for aspiration or pressure relief of gastric contents. A second orifice in the mask is used for ventilation. Hazards in the use of these tubes include trauma to the oesophagus and stomach, the risk of inducing vomiting and gastric rupture, and, paradoxically, unrecognised tracheal intubation.

Laryngeal mask airway

This recent development by Brain et al is an inflatable cuffed mask that is passed blindly into the hypopharynx to isolate the laryngeal inlet.[10] The mask is tolerated at a level of consciousness between that required for an oral airway and full intubation. Four sizes to fit infants to adults are available. It is important to check that the epiglottis does not fold back and obstruct the laryngeal opening in the mask during insertion. Although already popular in anaesthetic practice, their safety for an injured patient with a full stomach and risk of regurgitation or vomiting has yet to be evaluated.

1 Safar P, Bircher NG. Cardiopulmonary cerebral resuscitation. 3rd ed. London: WB Saunders, 1988:22-4.
2 Sellick BA. Cricoid pressure to control regurgitation of stomach contents during induction of anaesthesia. Lancet 1961;ii:404-6.
3 Howells TH. Disaster at the dining table. Br Med J 1984;289:511-2
4 Heimlich HJ. A lifesaving manoeuvre to prevent food choking. JAMA 1975;234:398-401.
5 Ferko JG III. Airtight advice. Emergency 1988;Jan:31-6.
6 Hamer M, Howells TH, Watson R. A survey of resuscitation ventilatory aids. Journal of the British Association for Immediate Care 1986;9:31-3.
7 Harrison RR, Maull KI, Keenan RL, Boyan CP. Mouth-to-mask ventilation: a superior method of rescue breathing. Ann Emerg Med 1982;11:74-6.
8 Nickalls RWD, Thomson CW. Mouth to mask respiration. Br Med J 1988;292:1350.
9 Seidelin PH, Stolarek IH, Littlewood DG. Comparison of six methods of emergency ventilation. Lancet 1986;ii:1274-5.
10 Brain AIJ, McGhee TD, McAteer EJ, Thomas A, Abu-Saad MAW, Bushman JA. The laryngeal mask airway. Development and preliminary trials of a new type of airway. Anaesthesia 1985;40:356-61.

ADVANCED LIFE SUPPORT IN GENERAL PRACTICE

BRIAN STEGGLES

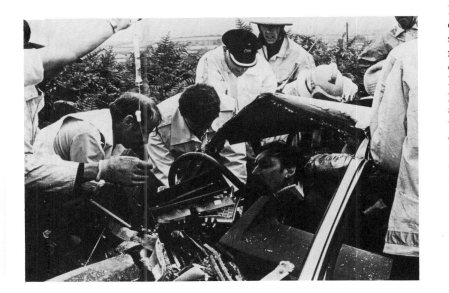

In 1990 the MRCGP examination will require candidates to show adequate skills in basic life support. These skills decay appreciably at six months, however, and regular retraining is essential. There is also no reason why advanced life support should not be provided by general practitioners, perhaps in combination with the ambulance service if appropriate, which would undoubtedly save many lives. The introduction of the diploma in immediate medical care at the Royal College of Surgeons of Edinburgh has established standards for prehospital emergency care and requires, as part of the practical assessment in the examination, that candidates show an ability in basic life support, defibrillation, and advanced airway care including intubation. These procedures are not difficult and could be taught easily at postgraduate centres, perhaps with the help of the hospital anaesthetic department for intubation training.

The life threatening emergencies occurring most commonly in general practice may be divided into three groups: cardiovascular, respiratory, and hypovolaemic. General practitioners may often be in a position to anticipate an emergency and so can either act to prevent it or be prepared to act immediately to correct it.

Cardiovascular emergencies

Every year in Britain half (about 60 000) the deaths from myocardial infarction occur before patients reach hospital. A general practitioner study showed that of the patients who died, 44% did so before the doctor arrived, 21% while the doctor was present, and a further 5% en route to hospital.[1] Hospital cardiac care units in the United Kingdom have substantially reduced their mortality after cardiac arrest, and in Seattle 35–40% of patients may survive prehospital ventricular fibrillation with paramedic defibrillation. In this country a general practitioner study of the use of defibrillators donated by the British Heart Foundation showed that nearly half the patients who suffered a cardiac arrest in the presence of doctors were resuscitated.[2]

The life saving potential of prehospital treatment after myocardial infarction is substantial—perhaps between 5000 and 6000 a year in this country. This can be achieved by:

(a) Improving the awareness and skills in cardiopulmonary resuscitation of the general public
(b) Training all doctors, nurses, and other staff in basic life support with regular refresher courses
(c) Introducing a chest pain policy for the surgery to reduce delays in response
(d) Doctors taking prompt action, including adequate pain relief
(e) Considering a dual response by a doctor and the ambulance service to any patient with chest pain
(f) Providing facilities for prehospital resuscitation including defibrillation.

Surgery policy

Reception staff to be aware of the importance of chest pain
All staff trained in basic life support
Register of patients at risk
Minimum delay in attending the call
If delay is likely consider mobilising ambulance first
or
Arrange dual response with the ambulance service for all coronary calls

---

Myocardial infarction

Action by doctor

Consider dual response
Establish intravenous route
Adequate pain relief to lessen risk of rhythm disturbance
Use intravenous *not* intramuscular morphine or diamorphine
Give aspirin
Consider maximum risk time and accompanying patient to hospital
Consider thrombolytics

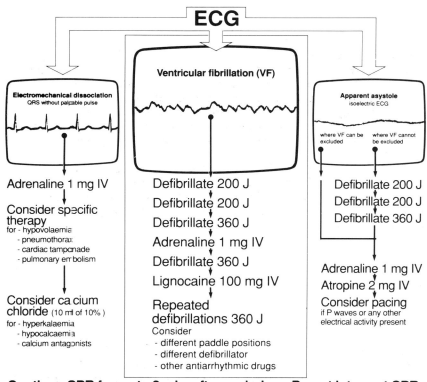

ECG

Ventricular fibrillation (VF)

Electromechanical dissociation
QRS without palpable pulse

Apparent asystole
isoelectric ECG

where VF can be excluded | where VF cannot be excluded

Adrenaline 1 mg IV

Consider specific therapy
for - hypovolaemia
- pneumothorax
- cardiac tamponade
- pulmonary embolism

Consider calcium chloride (10 ml of 10%)
for - hyperkalaemia
- hypocalcaemia
- calcium antagonists

Defibrillate 200 J
Defibrillate 200 J
Defibrillate 360 J
Adrenaline 1 mg IV
Defibrillate 360 J
Lignocaine 100 mg IV
Repeated defibrillations 360 J
Consider
- different paddle positions
- different defibrillator
- other antiarrhythmic drugs

Defibrillate 200 J
Defibrillate 200 J
Defibrillate 360 J

Adrenaline 1 mg IV
Atropine 2 mg IV
Consider pacing
if P waves or any other electrical activity present

Continue CPR for up to 2 min. after each drug. Do not interrupt CPR for more than 10 sec., except for defibrillation.
If an I.V. line cannot be established, consider giving double doses of adrenaline, lignocaine or atropine via an endotracheal tube.

Adequate pain relief reduces the risk of rhythm disturbances and thus the possibility of ventricular fibrillation. Morphine or diamorphine should be used and given *intravenously*—diluted in 10 ml water—and the dose titrated against the pain. Only if the intravenous route is impossible should an intramuscular injection be given, preferably into the deltoid muscle for most rapid absorption.

The commonest mechanism of cardiac arrest after myocardial infarction is ventricular fibrillation, which is potentially easily correctable with early defibrillation. Fewer than 15% of cardiac arrests occurring outside hospital are due to asystole or electromechanical dissociation, and these are considerably more difficult to treat successfully.

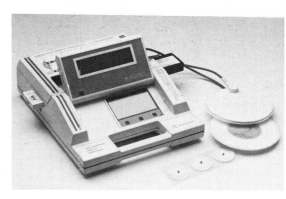

Semiautomatic or advisory defibrillator

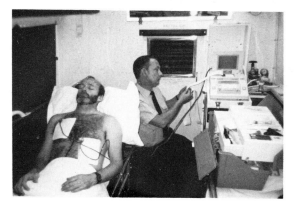

As it is impossible to predict which patients will develop ventricular fibrillation, or when, defibrillators should be available for all patients in the high risk period and from the time that the doctor or ambulance arrives until the patient reaches hospital. Many ambulance services now include cardiac care training, but few ambulance staff are yet trained in defibrillation. It may, however, be appropriate for the ambulance to carry a defibrillator and the doctor to be trained in using it, and for the dual response to be initiated for any patient with chest pain, whether they make primary contact with their doctor or with the ambulance service by 999 call. Ambulance response alone would mean that appropriate pain relief using morphine or diamorphine could not be given, and in some cases the crew would not be trained in cardiac care or defibrillation.

A report of the British Heart Foundation Working Group on the use of thrombolytic treatment in general practice supports this policy of dual response, the importance of speed and early pain relief, and the necessity for early administration of thrombolytic treatment.[3] There is, however, some hesitancy about the use of thrombolytics in the prehospital phase because of the associated risks of hypotension and the increased incidence of ventricular fibrillation. Both of these may be accentuated by the effects of vehicle movement, until more adequate information about their safety and efficacy is available thrombolytic treatment should be deferred until admission to hospital. The time to starting this treatment, however, should be as short as possible. In the absence of contraindications, aspirin may be given routinely as soon as possible to all patients diagnosed as experiencing acute myocardial infarction; the first dose of 150 mg should be crushed or chewed for quick absorption.

Other life threatening rhythm disturbances include ventricular tachycardia and bradycardia, which may require treatment immediately. The use of lignocaine infusion during transportation to hospital for other rhythm disturbances should be considered.

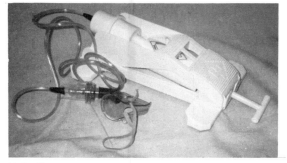

Nebuliser

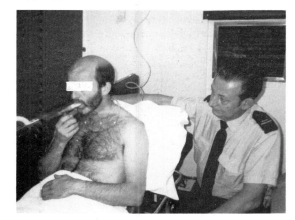

Intravenous infusion requirements

Intravenous cannulae
Drip set
Normal saline 2×500 ml
Haemaccel 1×500 ml
Fixing tape
Arm splint

Equipment

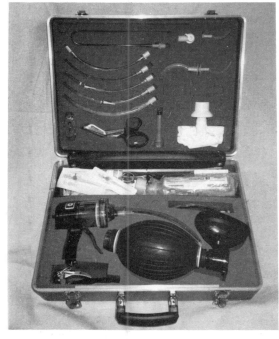

Resuscitation kit

Respiratory emergencies

The incidence of sudden death in severe asthma is increasing and it is important for patients and their relatives to be educated to understand the signs of severe deterioration of their condition. The appropriate use of nebulised or intravenous drugs by general practitioners in emergency is most important, and consideration needs to be given to the widespread use of nebulised drugs by the ambulance service.

Most cardiac arrests occurring in patients with asthma are secondary to hypoxia and asystole. Although these are more difficult to treat than ventricular fibrillation, the ability to intubate, ventilate with oxygen, and administer appropriate drugs may improve the chances of survival.

Hypovolaemia

Not all general practitioners wish to be associated with the emergency services in providing assistance at road accidents, but appreciable trauma on a lesser scale may occur at work or in the home, and profound hypovolaemia may result from such conditions as a bleeding peptic ulcer or antepartum haemorrhage. Lives can be saved by simple intravenous fluid replacement at the scene and en route to hospital.

It is always easier to take a drip down than to struggle to put one up later when the patient has become collapsed. The shocked patient who may need fluid replacement will benefit more if this is started early and continued during the journey to hospital, rather than waiting until arrival at the hospital. Restoring blood volume may be started with normal saline, up to one litre, followed by a plasma expander. Aggressive fluid replacement is often necessary and this must be appreciated. Fluid loss is probably the commonest cause of electromechanical dissociation seen before admission to hospital.

Putting up an intravenous line is no more difficult than taking blood. Choose a large and obvious vein, for example in the antecubital fossa. If the vein does not appear easily inflate a blood pressure cuff to a pressure between the systolic and diastolic levels.

Doctors associated with road accident care and participating in immediate care schemes and BASICS (British Association for Immediate Care) may decide to carry a considerable amount of equipment. For any other general practitioner a limited amount only is required, and each doctor should probably carry his own equipment in his car, as an emergency may occur at any time when he is away from the surgery. Several resuscitation kits that are not really expensive are produced, and advice about them may be obtained from BASICS.

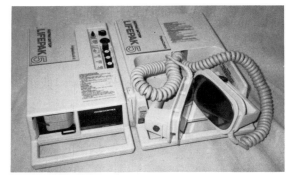

Manual defibrillator

Defibrillators

Some practices may wish to purchase their own defibrillator, although with their increasing provision in ambulances this may not always be necessary, particularly if the combined response of an ambulance and the doctor is considered when answering an emergency call to a suspected myocardial infarction. The British Heart Foundation will consider requests for help in buying defibrillators for general practitioners in areas where the ambulance service does not carry them or is too far away from the practice area for the necessary early intervention. Although earlier defibrillators were manually operated and required the operator to interpret the electrocardiagram, several advisory defibrillators are now available that analyse the rhythm automatically and prepare to deliver a shock to the patient if appropriate. They have high sensitivity and specificity for rhythm recognition, and training in the use of them is essentially simple and should take no more than four hours.

Drugs and dosages

Diamorphine 10 mg × 2 or morphine 20 mg* × 2
  (given slowly intravenously diluted with water
  to 10 ml and with antiemetic—titrate dose for
  pain relief)
Water for injection 10 ml × 2
Cyclizine 50 mg or metoclopramide 10 mg or
  prochlorperazine 12·5 mg (all may be mixed
  with diamorphine)
Naloxone 0·4 mg/ml ampoule × 2
Atropine sulphate 1 mg* × 2
Lignocaine 100 mg* in 5 ml (bolus)
         1000 mg* in 5 ml (infusion in 500 ml
            of normal saline)
Adrenaline 1 in 10 000—10 ml* × 2

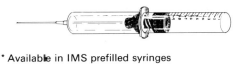

* Available in IMS prefilled syringes

Drugs

The essential drugs for advanced cardiac life support given in the Resuscitation Council guidelines are adrenaline, atropine, and lignocaine.[4] All are available in IMS prefilled syringes. Although emergency drugs should preferably be administered by the intravenous route, there are times, particularly in prehospital circumstances, when intravenous access may be difficult, and then endotracheal administration could be considered. Patients requiring these drugs have usually started undergoing a prolonged resuscitation attempt and will require the more secure and reliable endotracheal airway.

An anaphylactic shock drug kit (IMS), which contains 2 syringes of 1 in 10 000 adrenaline with instructions and dosages, is also available.

All general practitioners need to be trained to deal with emergencies. This must include basic life support as well as advanced cardiac life support, as there is no point in trying to progress to advanced care without adequate initiating and supporting basic care. Because skills decay, they must be regularly refreshed. The interrelation between general practitioners and the ambulance service needs to be considered further, particularly regarding the management of acute myocardial infarction.

Only by adopting these measures can the number of people who die from eminently treatable causes before reaching hospital be reduced.

Useful addresses
BASICS, 31c Lower Brook Street, Ipswich, Suffolk IP4 1AQ

IMS—International Medication Systems (UK) Ltd, 11 Royal Oak Way South, Daventry, Northamptonshire NN1 5PJ

I thank Laerdal Vitalograph, and Physio-Control for information about defibrillators.

1 Rawlins DC. Study of the management of suspected cardiac infarction by British immediate care doctors. Br Med J 1981;282:1677–9.
2 Colquhoun MC. Use of defibrillators by general practitioners. Br Med J 1988;297:335.
3 British Heart Foundation Working Group. Role of the general practitioner in managing patients with myocardial infarction: impact of thrombolytic treatment. Br Med J 1989;299:555–6.
4 Chamberlain DA. Advanced life support. Br Med J 1089;299:446–8.

RESUSCITATION BY AMBULANCE CREWS

RICHARD VINCENT

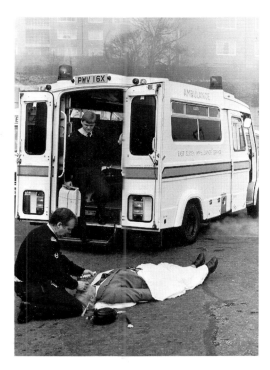

Sudden death outside hospital is common; in England alone more than 50 000 medically unattended deaths occur each year. The survival of countless victims of acute myocardial infarction, primary cardiac arrhythmia, trauma, or vascular catastrophe is threatened through lack of urgent care while they are remote from the skills and facilities of a hospital service. The case for providing prompt and effective resuscitation at the scene of an emergency is overwhelming, but only in the past few years has it begun to receive the attention it deserves.

Development of resuscitation ambulances

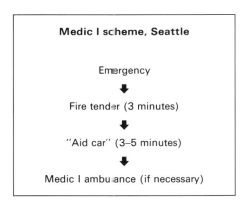

Medic I scheme, Seattle

Emergency
↓
Fire tender (3 minutes)
↓
"Aid car" (3–5 minutes)
↓
Medic I ambulance (if necessary)

The delivery of emergency care to patients before admission to hospital was pioneered in Europe in the late 1960s. Pilot schemes showed that resuscitation vehicles manned by *medical or nursing staff* could bring effective treatment to the victims of coronary disease or trauma.

The use of emergency vehicles carrying only *paramedic staff*—either in telephone contact with the hospital or acting entirely without supervision—was explored in the early 1970s, most extensively in the United States. Under the Medic I scheme started in Seattle in 1970 by Dr Leonard Cobb, the tenders of a highly coordinated fire service can reach an emergency in any part of the city within three minutes. All fire fighters are trained in basic life support and can call on secondary help from emergency medical technicians arriving in an "aid car" three to five minutes later. Third line support—well equipped Medic I Ambulances—are available for further assistance if required; they are crewed by paramedics who have received at least 12 months' full time training in emergency care. Seattle, with its now extensive community training programme in cardiopulmonary resuscitation as well as its paramedic force, remains an enviable example among schemes for the provision of prehospital care.

In the UK, the development of civilian paramedic schemes has been slow. The Brighton experiment in ambulance training began in 1971, and schemes in other centres followed independently over the next few years. But rapid progress in paramedic training has been hindered by the hesitation of hospital staff to accept the role of prehospital care and by the initial caution of the DHSS in supporting developments in this field. Moreover, because little additional remuneration has been given to crews for their extended skills and responsibility, and because until recently the ambulance service has focussed on transport rather than treatment, most of the progress in the past 15 years has resulted from individual enthusiasm for training and private donations for equipment. But the scene is changing rapidly. Widening clinical recognition and a growing acceptance by regulatory authorities of the value of prehospital care has led to the implementation of local resuscitation ambulance schemes in 79 health districts to date (see map).

Resuscitation ambulances manned by:
■ doctor or nurse
▨ ambulance staff only

Resuscitation ambulances in the United Kingdom

Data indicating the location of resuscitation ambulance crews in the UK were kindly made available by Dr Chamberlain on behalf of the British Cardiac Society and by Mrs Linda Bailey on behalf of the Trafford Centre for Medical Research.

Region	Health district
East Anglia	East Suffolk, Great Yarmouth and Waveney
Mersey	Chester,* Liverpool, Macclesfield,* St Helen and Knowsley, Wirral
NE Thames	Basildon and Thurrock, City and Hackney*
North Western	Burnley, Pendlebury and Rossendale, Bury, Lancaster, Preston,* Rochdale, South Manchester, Stockport, Tameside and Glossop
Northern	Darlington, Durham, East Cumbria, Hartlepool, North Tees,* NW Durham, Newcastle, North Tyneside, Northumberland, South Cumbria, South Tyneside, Sunderland, West Cumbria
Oxford	Aylesbury, East Berkshire, Kettering, Milton Keynes, West Berkshire, Wycombe
SE Thames	Brighton, Eastbourne, Hastings
SW Thames	Kingston and Esher, Mid Surrey, NW Surrey, SW Surrey, Worthing
South Western	Bristol and Weston, Cheltenham, Cornwall and Isles Of Scilly, Exeter, Frenchay, Gloucester, Torbay
Trent	Barnsley,* Bassetlaw, Central Nottinghamshire, Rotherham, South Derbyshire*
Wales	Clwyd, East Dyfed, Gwent, Gwynedd, South Glamorgan, West Glamorgan
Wessex	East Dorset, Swindon, West Dorset
West Midlands	Dudley,* Kidderminster and district, North Staffordshire, North Warwickshire, Sandwell, South Warwickshire, Walsall, Wolverhampton
Yorkshire	Airedale,* Hull,* Leeds Eastern, Leeds Western, Wakefield

* Manned by doctor or nurse. All others manned by ambulance staff only.

Training

In this country, paramedic training has varied widely between different pilot schemes; until recently there was no attempt at uniformity in the content, standard, duration, or organisation of training programmes, or in the evaluation or use of the skills of newly trained paramedics. All schemes have included instruction in basic life support and defibrillation. Training in intubation, infusion, and interpreting electrocardiograms has also been common, but less emphasis has been placed on the use of drugs and other emergency procedures.

More recently—after suggestions in the Miller Report (1966/7) and the recognition by the DHSS of the value of prehospital care—a national course for extended training in ambulance aid was launched by the National Staff Committee for ambulance staff in association with the NHS training authority. The NHS training authority course adds to the basic six week introductory tuition given to all ambulance staff and emphasises the extended skills of venous cannulation, recording and interpreting electrocardiograms, intubation, infusion, defibrillation, and optionally the use of selected drugs. The course is provided as an intensive nine week package, usually spread over several months. It covers the theoretical and practical knowledge needed for the extended care of various emergency conditions in a minimum instruction period of 320 hours. Some observers believe that the course in its present form cannot give the depth of knowledge or grounding provided by some earlier pilot schemes, and there may be advantages in a more modular pattern of tuition. But widespread acceptance and availability of the package, the system of accreditation with which it is associated, its more balanced syllabus to include non-cardiac emergencies, and its effect in promoting a growing interest in prehospital care should not be dismissed. The future may call for refinements in the delivery of instruction, but the NHS training authority course has done much to ensure that paramedic training in the UK has a future.

Drugs and routes of administration sanctioned for use by selected paramedics in the Brighton scheme

Drug	(Sub)-lingual	Intra-venous	Intra-muscular	Intra-cardiac	Endotracheal or via airway
Oxygen					x
Entonox					x
Nitroglycerine	x				x
Atropine		x	x		
Lignocaine		x	x		x
Adrenaline		x		x	x
Dexamethasone		x	x		
Naxolone		x			
Salbutamol					x
Haemaccel		x			
Glucagon		x	x		

Training in the use of drugs, as well as intracardiac cannulation and other advanced manoeuvres, remains controversial though experience in the Brighton scheme suggests that, with adequate training, paramedics may use various adjunctive techniques unsupervised to good effect and without harm. At the other end of the scale simple training for *all* ambulance staff in the use of *semiautomatic defibrillators* is undoubtedly worthwhile to rescue victims from the commonest reversible cause of cardiac death, ventricular fibrillation.

Retraining

Extended trained ambulance staff must undergo retraining or "refresher" periods, but the optimum timing, duration, and content of these has yet to be established. The NHS training authority package contains what is probably a minimum — three days in hospital every 9–15 months. Longer periods are likely to be more beneficial, and tailoring instruction to the experience of the individual paramedic would be welcomed. But any enhancement of refresher—or initial—training will demand noticeably more effort from ambulance and medical trainers.

Coordination and audit

Local enthusiasm remains a cornerstone for developing resuscitation ambulances. But a growing interest from the Department of Health and senior ambulance authorities is now leading to greater central encouragement and coordination. A newly formed advisory group, to be welcomed for its seniority and its multidisciplinary representation, is the Joint Colleges Ambulance Liaison Committee. Participants from the colleges of physicians, surgeons, anaesthetists, general practitioners, and nurses, and from the Regional Ambulance Officers Group, should together provide a strong voice setting prehospital care nationally on a sound medical and professional footing.

A growing interest in extended ambulance training has brought increasing pressure for audit. The first national extended training clinical audit was conducted from 1 January to 31 December 1988 by the National Ambulance Staff Committee associated with the NHS training authority. Its results were published in mid 1989. Of 68 questionnaires sent to ambulance authorities in the UK including the Channel Islands, 54 were returned, 47 of which indicated that extended trained skills are being practised in the region concerned. About 700 ambulance staff practise after training under the NHS training authority scheme, but more than 2000 others have come under some form of local instruction, if only in the use of cardiac monitoring. This first clinical audit provides an early, incomplete, but nevertheless unique insight into the use of extended skills in prehospital care. In the period studied over 28 000 patients received extended aid, including 4929 intubations and 4460 defibrillations carried out by ambulance staff.

Audit of extended aid in the UK during 1988

Extended aid practised in 47/68 (69%) regions

No of ambulance staff trained	2 700
Patients helped	28 000
Intubations	4 929
Defibrillations	4 460

Benefits of resuscitation ambulances

The observed benefits of a resuscitation ambulance service include:
- Reduction in delay to hospital admission
- Successful cardiopulmonary resuscitation
- Increased awareness of the need for rapid responses to emergencies
- Improved monitoring and support of the critically ill
- Improved standard of care for non-urgent cases

The delay in time to hospital admission and the yearly number of successful resuscitations are the easiest benefits to quantify. Rates at well established centres vary between 20 and 100 successful resuscitations each year for populations of about 350 000 (success means the subsequent discharge from hospital of a patient who is active and alert, but who would have stood no chance of survival without prehospital care). Techniques that aid comfort and prevent complications are less readily assessed, but cannot be dismissed.

Emergencies in which well trained paramedic crew can play vital part:

Life threatening arrhythmias
Respiratory arrest
Hypovolaemic shock
  internal haemorrhage
  trauma
Uncomplicated myocardial infarction
Severe left ventricular failure
Airway obstruction
Severe bronchospasm
Hypoglycaemic coma or pre-coma
Head injury
Drug overdose

Equipment for resuscitation ambulances

Defibrillator and monitor	Infusion box:		General box (contains
Sphygmomanometer	Hemaccel	4 × 500 ml	paramedics drugs box)
Intubation box:	Giving set		Syringes
Penlon laryngoscope	Selection of Venflons		Needles
Ambubag	Strapping tape		Venflons
Mask	Drugs box for paramedics:		Strapping
Jaw clamps	Lignocaine	4 × 5 ml 2%	Povidone spray
Magill forceps	Atropine	4 × 600 µg	Scissors
Endotracheal tubes 6, 7,	Adrenaline	4 × 10 ml 1:10 000	Sterile wipes
7·5, 8, 8·5, 9, 9·5 mm	Dexamethasone	2 × 400 µg	Razor and blades
10 ml syringes	Narcan	2 × 400 µg	Electrode jelly
Artery forceps	Salbutamol	2 × 2·5 mg	ECG leads
Adaptors	Sodium chloride	10 ml ampoules	Electrodes with straps
Connectors	Drugs box for doctors:		Defibrillator pads
Bandage	Calcium chloride	2 × 10 ml	Stethoscope
Lubricating jelly	Sodium bicarbonate	4 × 50 ml 0·4%	

Resuscitation ambulances and general practitioners

The working relationship between paramedic crews and general practitioners is for the most part amicable and productive. Most general practitioners welcome the facilities offered by a resuscitation ambulance service and often speak highly of the individual performances of paramedics at the scene of an emergency. Many admit that the skills of paramedics in dealing with life threatening conditions—and occasionally the equipment carried by the resuscitation ambulance—complement their own. Any conflicts that have arisen usually reflect overenthusiasm of the trained ambulance staff; misunderstandings can usually be resolved by mutual discussion with the senior hospital staff overseeing the scheme.

A new dimension in this relationship is possible since the advent of thrombolytic treatment for acute myocardial infarction. The dramatic effect of thrombolysis in improving the outcome of a heart attack is most noticeable when treatment is given soon after the onset of major symptoms. But the potentially serious side effects of thrombolytic treatment dictate that it is used with care and only when the diagnosis is at least reasonably certain. The use of thrombolytic agents by ambulance staff (who may reach patients rapidly but who have limited diagnostic expertise) or by general practitioners (whose diagnostic skill is greater but who may not be able to get to patients so soon) is an idea to be approached with caution. The mechanics and merits of prehospital thrombolysis must be evaluated before any widespread recommendations can be made, but collaboration between ambulance staff and general practitioners in the early management of patients with acute myocardial infarction—with a view to early thrombolysis—should be strengthened.

Strategy for resuscitation and prehospital care

Relationships between hospitals, general practitioners, ambulance staff, and members of the community

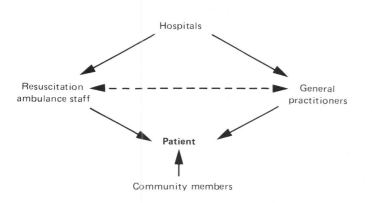

Resuscitation ambulances should be regarded as one important part of a strategic pattern for emergency care in the community; the hospital, the general practitioner, and the community itself make equally important contributions to the optimum treatment of the injured or seriously ill. The hospital service provides not only the facilities for continuing patient care but a resource for training, encouragement, review, and in some centres research in simple and advanced resuscitation techniques. The role of the community can be vital. Even with a rapidly responsive and well drilled paramedic service, delay is inevitable between a 999 call and the arrival of the resuscitation ambulance; in circulatory arrest this delay may be crucial. Bystander cardiopulmonary resuscitation in the vulnerable few minutes before the ambulance arrives has been shown to bring an appreciable improvement in the short and long term outcome of prehospital care.

The future

Two important factors give optimism for rapid growth in resuscitation ambulances: an increasing interest in advanced training by the National Staff Committee and other central bodies, and the enthusiasm of ambulance staff themselves for paramedic training. But these factors alone are insufficient: vision and commitment by senior medical staff are mandatory if local facilities for prehospital care are to be established and maintained, and if lives are to be saved by skills that can be learned and applied effectively by ambulance staff.

RESUSCITATION IN THE ACCIDENT AND EMERGENCY DEPARTMENT

ANDREW K MARSDEN, ALASTAIR McGOWAN

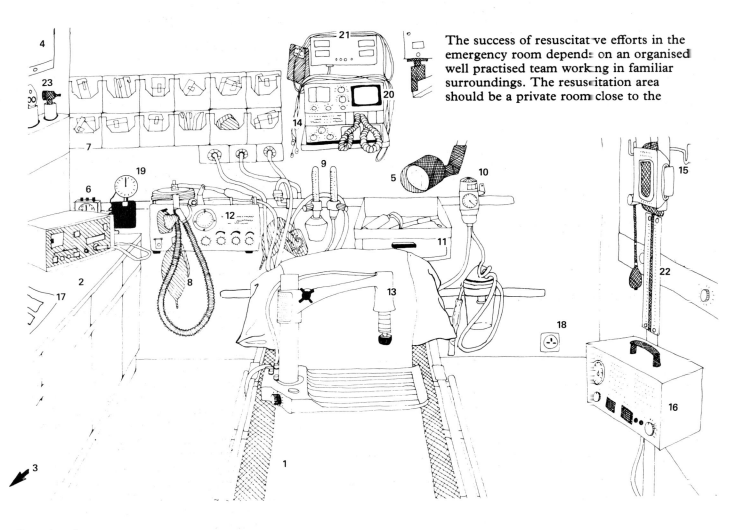

The success of resuscitative efforts in the emergency room depends on an organised well practised team working in familiar surroundings. The resuscitation area should be a private room close to the

General equipment
(1) Patient trolly, variable height and tilt; rigid mattress; oxygen, suction drip poles, etc
(2) Work unit with disposables storage under
(3) Procedures trolley
(4) X ray viewer
(5) High intensity spotlamp
(6) Stop clock
(Not shown: scrub basin, refuse bin)

Airway and breathing equipment
(7) Storage for tubes, airway, masks, etc
(8) Bag valve mask unit
(9) Oxygen therapy equipment
(10) Suction unit
(11) Intubation equipment
(12) Automatic ventilator

Circulation equipment
(13) Pneumatic chest compressor
(14) External defibrillator-pacemaker
(15) Drip stand with pressure infuser
(16) Blood warmer
(17) Resuscitation drugs
(Not shown: antishock trousers)

Diagnostic and monitoring equipment
(18) Socket for portable x ray or image intensifier
(19) Sphygmomanometer
(20) ECG monitor
(21) Automatic blood pressure and temperature monitor
(22) Central venous pressure monitor
(23) Otoscope and ophthalmoscope

emergency entrance at least 23·5 m^2 (250 ft^2) with piped gases, wash hand basin, good lighting, and x ray power points as essential fittings. Operative surgical facilities should be close by.

Doctor 1

Overall charge. Dictates priorities.
Airway control, intubation/ventilation
Observes conscious level
Determines referral
? Central venous pressure

Nurse A

Prepares resuscitation room
Assists doctor 1 then doctor 2
Applies monitoring leads
Draws up and charts drugs
Sets up for special procedures

Doctor 3

First intravenous cross match
Splints legs
Assists doctor 2

Doctor 2

Examines chest,
abdomen, limbs
? 2nd Intravenous line
? Chest drain
? Peritoneal lavage
? Urinary catheter
Completes notes

Nurse B

Assists doctor 3
Supervises infusion
Charts fluids
Records pulse,
blood pressure, etc

All staff help undress patient

Resuscitation room positions
(after Davidson)

II Airway Ventilation Intubation

III

External chest
compression
Checks pulse

(V Operates defibrillator)

IV

Intravenous infusion
Administers and records
drugs
Withdraws blood gases

I Leader

Supervises and directs team
Diagnoses cardiac rhythms
Controls treatment
Arranges after care

Organisation of cardiac
resuscitation (the megacode)

Forewarning will usually be from the ambulance service by telephone or, increasingly, via a two way radio call.

Medical and nursing staff take up their positions around the patient according to a preagreed scheme.[1] All staff help to undress the patient. There should be a readily apparent leader from among the senior medical staff who will direct the team, prescribe treatments, and decide aftercare. One doctor will stay with the patient and be responsible for the medical care, assessment, and records of the patient. The division of duties will vary according to whether the episode is medical, surgical, or traumatic. The megacode approach, using an ordered team of four, is recommended in cardiorespiratory arrest.[2]

The following scheme relates to the resuscitation of an unconscious casualty (for further discussion about resuscitating multiply injured patients see the next chapter). The principles are, however, fundamental to any type of emergency and are as follows.

(1) Assume a spinal cord lesion until proved otherwise. All neck movements kept to a minimum until the integrity of the cervical spine has been shown radiographically.

(2) Staunch obvious gross external haemorrhage by direct pressure over the bleeding point and raising of the affected part.

(3) Cover and seal any open (sucking) chest wounds.

(4) *Airway*
Establish and maintain a clear airway. This will include postural methods; aspiration of blood, mucus, vomit, etc, with a sucker; and, definitively, the passage of a cuffed endotracheal tube. A tongue support such as the oropharyngeal or nasopharyngeal tube airway may be useful. When there is total obstruction of the upper airway—for example, from oedema or inflammation at the vocal cords—a laryngotomy through the cricothyroid membrane may be necessary. This technique is safer in inexpert hands in an emergency than the more elective procedure of tracheostomy.

(5) *Breathing*
A chest radiograph and blood gas analysis will be required early in the assessment of all chest emergencies. Ventilate for apnoea or respiratory inadequacy: aim to keep the arterial oxygen pressure above 10 kPa and the carbon dioxide below 5.5 kPa. This may be achieved by a bag valve mask device with added oxygen. With such a device the "feel" of the compliance may

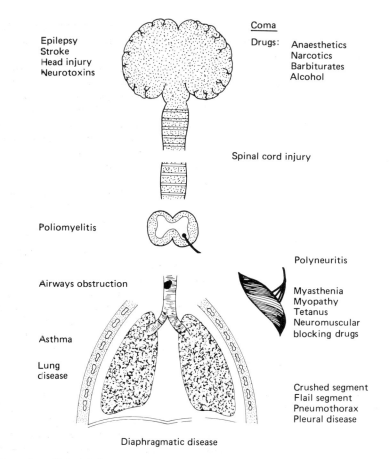

Coma

Epilepsy
Stroke
Head injury
Neurotoxins

Drugs: Anaesthetics
Narcotics
Barbiturates
Alcohol

Spinal cord injury

Poliomyelitis

Polyneuritis

Airways obstruction

Myasthenia
Myopathy
Tetanus
Neuromuscular
blocking drugs

Asthma

Lung
disease

Crushed segment
Flail segment
Pneumothorax
Pleural disease

Diaphragmatic disease

Causes of ventilatory failure

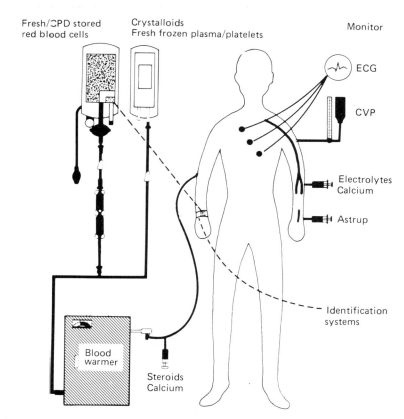

Safer blood transfusion

give clues about the presence of remediable problems within the chest, such as a tension pneumothorax (an important cause of cardiorespiratory collapse in acute asthma), flail segment, or lung contusion.

Full thickness circumferential burns of neck and chest require escharotomy to release restriction of chest wall movement. Inequality of ventilation may indicate inadvertent intubation of the right main bronchus or a major air leak within the tracheobronchial tree. Chest drainage is indicated on the side of a flail segment, in the presence of surgical emphysema, or if there is a traumatic pneumothorax, however small. All pneumothoraces must be drained before ventilation. If given early high dose corticosteroids—for example, methylprednisolone 30 mg/kg intravenously—may be of advantage in blast lung injury, lung contusion, near drowning, and smoke inhalation.

(6) Circulation

Support the circulation by ensuring secure venous access with the largest cannula size achievable in a reliable vein. The antecubital fossae are, perhaps, the best sites for intravenous infusion in major trauma, but a central vein, such as the internal jugular, may need to be catheterised for fluid push or central venous pressure monitoring. In profound shock consider the use of the saphenous vein in the groin accessed by cutting down at the saphenofemoral junction. Blood samples will be withdrawn for grouping and cross matching, haemoglobin and packed cell volume estimations, and analysis of electrolyte, urea, and glucose concentrations.

For profound shock of whatever cause the volume of the transfused fluid is more important than content. As a general principle in severe traumatic shock type specific blood is preferred, with attention given to the multiplicity of problems of blood transfusion. If more than eight units of blood need to be given fresh frozen plasma, platelets, calcium gluconate, and a clotting screen may be required.

Haemorrhagic shock cannot be successfully managed unless the bleeding is brought under control and blood loss replaced—and this may require immediate surgery. The application of antishock trousers may control haemorrhage from the abdomen, pelvis, or legs, for example in stabilising patients exsanguinating from a ruptured aortic aneurysm. The release of this device should be under strict surgical control in the operating theatre.

In cardiac arrest due to hypovolaemia, especially as a result of penetrating injury, the treatment should be immediate thoracotomy (to allow internal cardiac massage and cross clamping of the aorta) and blood replacement.

(7) Establish baseline monitoring and start observations of pulse, respiratory rate, blood pressure, and central venous pressure when appropriate. Monitor the electrocardiagram and the oxygen saturation if a pulse oximeter is available. Except when there is blood at the urethral meatus, a urinary catheter should be inserted and the urine output measured. Observations of the level of consciousness, using an approved coma scale, pupillary responses, and limb movements should be charted every 15 minutes. A breath or blood alcohol assessment may be valuable.

(8) The victim should be examined fully, front and back and from head to toe. Up to 30% of fractures are not recognised in the resuscitation room.[3] Radiographs of the skull, cervical spine, chest, and pelvis should be routinely obtained in the multiply injured patient. Peritoneal lavage should be considered in the diagnosis of intra-abdominal haemorrhage in casualties who are comatose or paralysed or who have injury to both chest and pelvis. Computerised diagnostic ultrasound (the "midliner") is a valuable and inexpensive screening test for intracranial haematoma.[4]

(9) If the level of consciousness is deteriorating obtain immediate neurosurgical advice. Mannitol 20% 1 g/kg effectively lowers intracranial pressure in the short term. Its use, together with paralysis and hyperventilation, is best confined to patients who have been accepted for neurosurgery. Convulsions should be brought under control with titrations of intravenous diazepam. Check for hypoglycaemia as a contributory factor.

(10) Administer human antitetanus immunoglobulin unless tetanus prophylaxis is known to be up to date.

(11) Organise a diagnosis list and scale of priorities for subsequent care. Arrange referral to the specialty or specialties most urgently concerned and ensure that responsibility for the care of the whole patient is undertaken by an identifiable consultant whose firm will organise the involvement of other specialties as needed. Arrange safe, controlled transit of the patient to theatre, investigation room, or ward and the transfer of responsibility thereafter.

At the conclusion of resuscitation each member of the team should take part in the cleaning up that invariably takes place. Records should be completed, equipment and drugs should be rechecked and replaced, and, some time later, a private, informal "debriefing" is valuable in assessing the procedures and identifying any errors and scope for improvement.

A relatives' room is an essential part of the accident and emergency department.[5] The fears and uncertainties of relatives should be allayed whenever possible. The breaking of tragic news, a difficult and unpleasant duty, is the responsibility of the senior doctor present in the company of the senior nurse.

Emergency department resuscitation, though infrequent, is demanding and exciting. Perhaps only 1% of cases presented to the accident and emergency department (one or two a day) require the use of the resuscitation room.[6] Thorough planning, organisation, and team effort make such cases particularly rewarding.

1 Davison HA. Resuscitation room routine. *British Journal of Accident Emergency Medicine* 1983;1:15–16.
2 Kaye W, Linhares KC, Breault RV, Norris PA, Stamoulis CC, Khan AH. The mega-code for training the advanced cardiac life support team. *Heart and Lung* 1981;10:860–5.
3 McClaren CA, Robertson CE, Little K. Missed orthopaedic injuries in the resuscitation room. *J Roy Coll Surg Edinb* 1983;20:399–10.
4 Price DJ. Computerised ultrasound for the monitoring of head injured patients. *Intensive Care World* 1985;2:88–91.
5 Wilson DH. Every emergency department should have one—an interview room. *Br Med J* 1976;i:87–8.
6 Potter BT, Howie CR, Brooks SC, *et al*. The use of a resuscitation room: a review of current trends. *Injury* 1985;14:461–4.

RESUSCITATION OF MULTIPLY INJURED PATIENTS

ANDREW K MARSDEN

Experience of the advanced trauma life support system of the American College of Surgeons has highlighted the value of a structured approach to resuscitating multiply injured patients within the first "golden hour" after injury. The advanced trauma life support programme has now been adopted under licence by the Royal College of Surgeons of England for widespread dissemination within the United Kingdom. The approach is prescriptive and didactic and may be criticised by the British practitioner. The dogma of advanced trauma life support, however, is surely its main merit; safe and successful resuscitation is more likely when prejudices are abandoned and the protocol followed to the letter.

The advanced trauma life support scheme has four components: primary survey, resuscitation phase, secondary survey, and definitive care phase. The primary survey includes simultaneous attention to the ABCs:

A Airway maintenance and control of the cervical spine,
B Breathing and ventilation,
C Circulation and control of haemorrhage,
D Disability and neurological state,
E Exposure by completely undressing the patient.

During the resuscitation phase oxygenation is reassessed and haemorrhage controlled. Attention is given to life threatening conditions, such as tension pneumothorax, identified in the primary survey.

This chapter is a précis of the main steps outlined in the primary survey and resuscitation phases of the advanced trauma life support protocol.

> **Advanced trauma life support**
>
> Four components:
>   primary survey
>   resuscitation phase
>   secondary survey
>   definitive care phase

> **ABCs of the primary survey**
>
> A airway maintenance and control of cervical spine
> B breathing and ventilation
> C circulation and control of haemorrhage
> D disability and neurological state
> E exposure by completely undressing patient

Assume a spinal injury until proved otherwise

In line cervical stabilisation

Any patient with multisystem trauma, especially blunt injury above the clavicle, is at risk from the possibility of a cervical spine fracture. Excessive neck movement can convert a fracture without neurological damage into an injury with neurological damage. The patient's head and neck should not be hyperextended or hyperflexed to establish or maintain an airway.

In line cervical immobilisation should be maintained until an adequate lateral radiograph of the cervical spine (showing all cervical vertebrae and the interface between C7 and T1) has been obtained and passed as normal.

Airway care

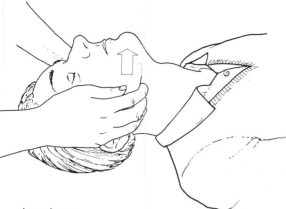

Jaw thrust

Initial attempts to open the airway in an unconscious victim of trauma include the chin lift and jaw thrust manoeuvres. The head tilt procedure should be avoided in multiply injured patients.

Obvious mucus, vomit, and blood should be removed with a sucker.

A tongue support such as the oropharyngeal or nasopharyngeal tube airway may be useful.

Securing the airway by the passage of a cuffed endotracheal tube is important to prevent the inhalation of regurgitated stomach contents and to permit effective ventilation. If there is no immediate need for endotracheal intubation a cervical spine radiograph should be obtained next. If the immediate need for an airway precludes radiography of the cervical spine, and if the patient is breathing, nasotracheal intubation should be attempted. If the patient is apnoeic orotracheal intubation with in line cervical immobilisation should be attempted. The intubation procedure should be preceeded by a moment's oxygenation and ventilation.

Needle and surgical cricothyroidotomy

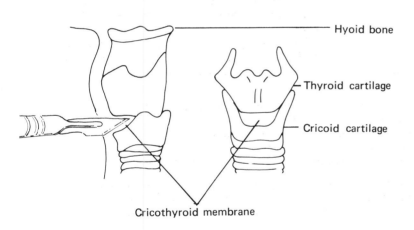

Hyoid bone

Thyroid cartilage

Cricoid cartilage

Cricothyroid membrane

Cricothyroidotomy or laryngotomy

If the upper airway is obstructed (by glottic oedema, laryngeal injury, or severe oropharyngeal trauma) and the doctor is unable to intubate the trachea then a surgical airway is required. A surgical opening into the cricothyroid membrane is ideal, but in unskilled hands inserting a needle into the cricothyroid membrane or into the trachea below the obstruction is an acceptable alternative. The latter is preferable for a child aged under 12.

Needle cricothyroidotomy may be combined with jet insufflation of the lungs to provide adequate ventilation for up to 45 minutes while more formal airway control is established. Jet insufflation is achieved by puncturing the trachea with a 12 or 14 gauge intravenous needle whose cannula is connected to an oxygen source at 15 litres a minute with either a Y connector or a side hole cut in the delivery tubing; intermittent ventilation is obtained by covering and releasing the open hole with the thumb, one second on and four seconds off.

The technique of surgical cricothyroidotomy is to make a skin incision through the cricothyroid membrane and dilate the opening with a curved haemostat so that a small endotracheal tube or a 5 to 7 mm tracheostomy tube can be inserted.

Oxygenation and ventilation

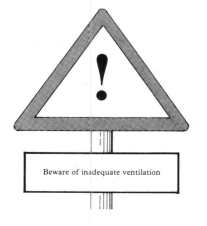

Beware of inadequate ventilation

It does not follow that, because the airway is clear, the breathing is adequate. The patient's chest should be exposed to check for adequacy of respiratory movements and the lungs auscultated for adequate air entry to all areas. A respiratory rate of more than 20 breaths a minute suggests respiratory compromise; the most common traumatic causes of respiratory inadequacy are tension pneumothorax, open pneumothorax, and large flail chest with pulmonary contusion.

The oxygen delivery system should be capable of permitting a fractional inspired oxygen of at least 85%, which cannot be provided with a simple face mask or nasal prongs. Instead, a tight fitting oxygen reservoir face mask should be used with a high oxygen flow rate of at least 12 litres a minute.

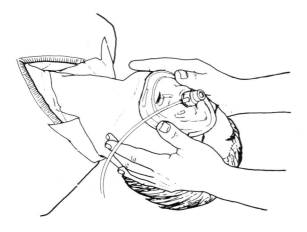

Until the patient's condition is stable, ventilation should be performed with a bag valve mask device or with a mouth to face mask system. For ventilation by one rescuer, mouth to mask ventilation has been shown to be more effective and is preferred.

A patient deteriorating rapidly from tension pneumothorax should undergo thoracentesis. To relieve the pneumothorax a 12 or 14 gauge over the needle catheter, preferably "valved" by attachment to a syringe containing saline, is inserted into the pleural cavity in the second intercostal space in the mid clavicular line. Once the circulation has been assessed and stabilised a chest tube will need to be inserted.

Circulation

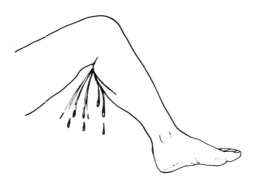

Obvious external haemorrhage should be identified and controlled using direct pressure on the wound. Haemostats and tourniquets are potentially dangerous and should not normally be used. Appropriate application of a pneumatic antishock garment might be useful in temporarily controlling major bleeding from the abdomen, pelvis, or legs.

Any hypotension after injury must be assumed to be due to hypovolaemia until proved otherwise. The state of the circulation is rapidly assessed by observing the degree of consciousness, the skin colour, and the pulse. When unconsciousness has resulted from haemorrhage at least 50% of the blood can be assumed to have been lost. Similarly, an ashen grey skin of the face coupled with the pallor of exsanguinated limbs imply a blood loss of at least 30%. The pulse rate and regularity correlate well with the degree of haemorrhagic shock; the loss of the central pulse at one or more sites suggests cardiac compromise and impending cardiac arrest.

Access to the circulation should be established with at least two large bore intravenous catheters, such as 16 or 14 gauge intravenous lines, in each antecubital fossa. Blood should be withdrawn for grouping and base line laboratory studies.

The choice and method of intravenous fluid replacement is contentious. That recommended in the advanced trauma life support programme is an initial rapid infusion of a balanced salt solution of up to two or three litres. Thereafter type specific whole blood is given while cross matched blood is being prepared. In life threatening haemorrhage, unmatched but type specific blood is used in preference to type O blood.

Sign (skin colour, degree of consciousness, and pulse)	State of circulation
Ashen grey face and pale limbs	30% blood loss
Unconscious	50% blood loss
No central pulse at one or more site	Possible cardiac compromise or impending arrest

Neurological assessment

Level of response
A alert
V responds to vocal stimuli
P responds to painful stimuli
U unresponsive

As part of the primary survey, the patient's level of consciousness is assessed and pupillary size and reaction measured. A quick check of the level of response can be given by use of the AVPU mnemonic:

A alert,
V responds to vocal stimuli,
P responds to painful stimuli,
U unresponsive.

A more detailed assessment should be carried out subsequently using the Glasgow coma scale, which enables the revised trauma score to be calculated.

Monitoring

Glasgow coma scale

Eye opening	Best motor response	Best verbal response
4 Spontaneous	6 Obeys commands	5 Oriented
3 To speech	5 Localises pain	4 Confused
2 To pain	4 Flexes to pain	3 Inappropriate
1 None	3 Abnormal flexion	2 Incomprehensible
	2 Extension	1 None
	1 None	

Maximum total score 15

Revised trauma score

Glasgow coma score	Systolic blood pressure	Respiratory rate	Coded value for each variable
13–15	>90	10–29	4
9–12	76–89	>29	3
6–8	50–75	6– 9	2
4–5	1–49	1– 5	1
3	0	0	0

Maximum total score 12

During the resuscitation phase the patient's condition will be closely monitored and, in particular, specific improvements will be sought in the pulse, blood pressure, pulse pressure, ventilatory rate, arterial blood gas concentrations, and urinary output. The electrocardiogram should be monitored. Unless there are specific injuries contraindicating it, a urinary catheter and a gastric tube should be inserted.

The procedures outlined in this chapter are the minimum necessary to identify life threatening problems and provide initial resuscitation. Although a firm plan of action can often be based on the initial phases of primary survey and resuscitation, the detailed early assessment of a multiply injured patient is incomplete without a full secondary survey and attention to specific problems.

Details of advanced trauma life support courses and training may be obtained from the Royal College of Surgeons, Lincolns Inn Fields, London.

RESUSCITATION IN HOSPITAL
T R EVANS

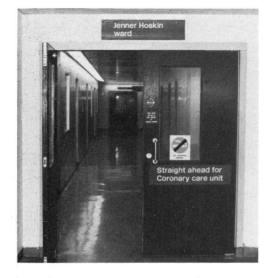

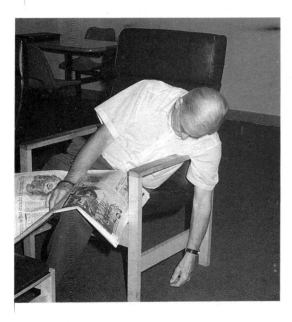

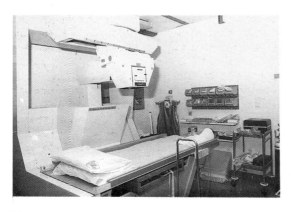

In hospital it is important to consider the areas where resuscitation may be required because the logistics of delivery vary between areas.

Intensive care areas—In the intensive care unit, accident and emergency department, coronary care unit, anaesthetic rooms and operating theatres, and special care baby units skilled personnel with appropriate equipment should be readily available to start advanced life support immediately. Most patients will be monitored and many will have established intravenous lines. The number of successful resuscitations in these areas should provide an example to the rest of the hospital, as should the skill in resuscitation shown by their staff.

General wards—Here varying degrees of nursing and medical skill and equipment may be available. The emphasis has to be on immediate basic life support, usually by nursing staff, with the cardiac arrest team being summoned to provide advanced life support. Basic life support should be taught to all ward staff; they should appreciate that effective basic life support procedures are essential until the cardiac arrest team arrives and that the survival of patients is greatly affected by the speed at which basic support is started and the adequacy with which it is maintained.

Non-ward areas—In x ray, radiotherapy, physiotherapy, nuclear medicine departments, etc, the emphasis is again on basic life support until the cardiac arrest team arrives. In the past very little effort has been made to train paramedical staff, such as physiotherapists, radiographers, and medical physicists in basic life support, or even to explain to them how the cardiac arrest call system works. If properly trained there is no reason why they cannot apply adequate basic life support until the team arrives.

Other areas where the patient may attend adjacent to the hospital include psychiatric day hospitals and facilities for the physically or mentally handicapped. Again all attending staff should be taught basic life support and there should be a well rehearsed procedure for them to summon help, whether it be the cardiac arrest team if they are within the confines of the hospital or an ambulance if they are too far removed.

General thoroughfares of the hospital—basic life support should be provided by any staff available. Ideally any person working in a hospital should be able to provide basic life support, so training should ultimately be extended to all grades and categories, to include such groups as clerical, administrative, and portering staff. Obviously they must know how to alert the hospital cardiac arrest team, and the patient will then usually be removed to the nearest clinical area for treatment unless the necessary equipment can be brought to the patient.

Clearly, only in the intensive care areas will advanced life support be started immediately. In a well run intensive care or coronary care unit it is reasonable to expect the nursing staff to have resuscitated many of the patients, especially those in ventricular fibrillation, well before the doctors arrive.

In all other areas the staff on the spot must immediately initiate adequate basic life support and maintain it until the cardiac arrest team arrives. In these areas the start of advanced life support may be delayed by four to five minutes or more because in most hospitals patients on the open ward and other areas are not monitored and the nurses are not specially trained or allowed to defibrillate and have no equipment immediately available except for airway equipment. They will have to dial an emergency telephone number, which should be marked on every telephone, and be taught to give a clear message stating the exact location of the cardiac or respiratory arrest.

If there are enough people to apply basic life support other members of staff should position themselves so that they can direct the cardiac arrest team immediately to the patient.

Cardiac arrest team

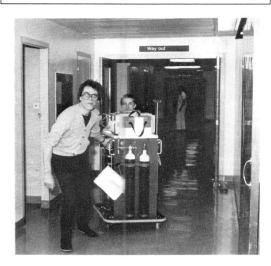

Cardiac arrest team

(1) Generally: duty medical and anaesthetic registrars
   senior house officer
   senior nurse(s)
   porter and trolley
(2) Team needs bleeps with speech channel
(3) Operator tells team location of arrest. Repeats message
(4) If message not clear team member rings operator: makes it clear not another arrest call
(5) Doctors and porter need keys to commandeer lift

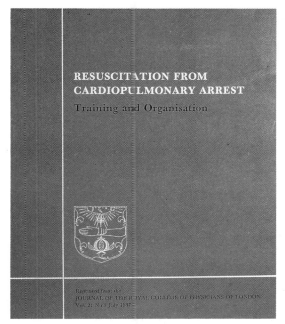

In many hospitals the cardiac arrest team consists of the duty medical and anaesthetic registrars, a more junior doctor, one or two senior nurses, and a porter who will bring the emergency trolley. All will carry special bleeps which will be simultaneously alerted by the switchboard operator in case of cardiac arrest. These bleeps should have a speech channel so that the operator can give the location of the emergency. The operator should speak slowly and clearly and repeat the message at least once—for example, "Tavistock ward—third floor, north block." If the message is not clearly understood by any member of the cardiac arrest team he or she should dial the emergency number and speak directly to the operator, making it clear that the inquiry is about the location of the cardiac arrest and not a second cardiac arrest call. In multistorey hospitals special emergency keys to the lifts should be provided for the two senior doctors and the porter with the emergency trolley to enable them to commandeer the nearest lift and reach the patient as soon as possible.

Until the team arrives basic life support with expired air respiration (with or without the use of an airway or mask or ventilation using a face mask and a self inflating bag) must be provided. If patients are known to be suffering from contagious diseases an airway or face mask with a non-returnable valve must be used.

In many ways the situation in non-intensive care areas is identical to a cardiac arrest in the street in a city where emergency medical technicians or paramedic crews have a very rapid response time of three or five minutes such as in Seattle, Washington State. If the ward staff can maintain basic life support effectively until the arrest team arrives hospital discharge rates would be much higher. The Seattle figures suggest that 30% of patients who receive bystander basic life support are defibrillated outside hospital and survive to leave hospital. As the aetiology of cardiac arrest in hospitals is often more complicated the survival figures would probably be lower, but the concept remains the same.

Everyone concerned in hospital resuscitation must be prepared and properly trained. A cardiac arrest call must initiate a well rehearsed, well orchestrated sequence of events—much the same as action stations being called on a warship.

Resuscitation panel

RESUSCITATION FROM CARDIOPULMONARY ARREST
Training and Organisation

Reprinted from the JOURNAL OF THE ROYAL COLLEGE OF PHYSICIANS OF LONDON Vol. 21 No. 3 July 1987

Each hospital should have a subcommittee or panel, meeting at least quarterly to discuss problems and general policies. It should report directly to the hospital medical executive committee. The subcommittee should include senior and junior hospital doctors, nurses, pharmacists, the infectious diseases control officer, technicians, and an administrator and should have the power to co-opt or invite to meetings anyone with special knowledge or who has a particular problem to discuss. The problem may be one of communications because of bleep black spots, there may be lift problems, or there may be problems of standardising drugs or equipment. The resuscitation protocols for both basic and advanced life support must be displayed throughout the hospital and taught by the resuscitation training officer and medical and nursing staff. All hospitals should implement the 1987 Royal College of Physicians report, *Cardiopulmonary resuscitation: training and organisation*. The final chapter discusses the ethics of resuscitation, and one of the duties of the subcommittee is to remind senior doctors of their responsibilities. Any patient of any age or suffering from any disease will rightly be subjected to an attempt at resuscitation unless a contrary instruction has been left by the medical staff and entered into the medical and nursing records.

Resuscitation training officer

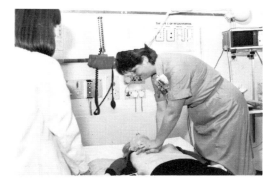

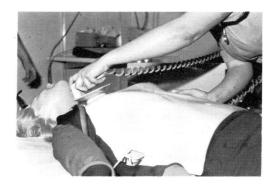

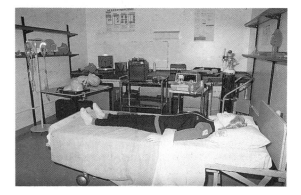

All hospitals need a designated person responsible for training staff in basic and advanced cardiopulmonary resuscitation. The resuscitation training officer should organise and document training courses, take care of training equipment, and audit cardiac arrest calls. A suitable person would have had extensive experience in resuscitation either as a sister or charge nurse or as a paramedic in the ambulance service. The officer should be responsible to one or two consultants on the resuscitation subcommittee but is expected to act independently.

Included in the training programme are all junior medical staff, any medical students, all trained nurses, paramedical staff such as physiotherapists, ancillary staff, and, probably in future, ambulance crews and even the lay public.

Once staff become aware of the availability of such courses it becomes difficult for training officers to find enough time to teach all staff personally and they will have to delegate some of the work. At our hospital the teaching of the student nurses is shared with the teaching staff of the school of nursing. This should ensure uniformity of teaching from the time a nurse starts training in the hospital to the time he or she achieves a more senior appointment.

Most hospitals no longer have a regular rotation of nursing staff between day and night duty and therefore before the training officer has to spend some time on night duty training at least the senior night staff in areas where cardiac arrests are likely to occur. Also if nights are not worked any logistical problems peculiar to cardiac arrests occurring at night will not be identified.

In future we hope that the training officer will train groups of instructors who will continually be subject to retraining and revision and these instructors will teach other members of staff. Larger hospitals may need more than one training officer.

Retention of resuscitation skills is known to be poor. There is no substitute for teaching on proper manikins, and the major part of any training session should be devoted to manikin practice. Training in resuscitation and the range of manikins and models available are reviewed in subsequent chapters. Because of the time taken to set all the equipment up and arrange a simulated cardiac arrest, it is important that the hospital should have a designated room for resuscitation training.

It is to be hoped that in future no doctor or nurse will qualify who cannot perform adequate basic life support. Hospitals and perhaps community bases will provide regular revision courses. For those who need to practise advanced life support the hospital will arrange proper training and retraining. Accreditation of posts should include evaluation of resuscitation practice and training procedures.

POSTRESUSCITATION CARE

A D REDMOND

Full recovery from cardiac arrest is rarely immediate. The restoration of electrocardiographic complexes marks the start and not the end of a successful resuscitation. The true end point is a fully conscious, neurologically intact patient with a spontaneous stable cardiac rhythm and an adequate urine output.

The chances of achieving this are greatly enhanced if the conditions in the box are met.

Once spontaneous cardiac output has been restored ensure that a senior doctor is summoned and makes a decision about transferring the patient to an intensive care area. Elective ventilation is often necessary and such decisions require experience and authority. Clearly if the time from the onset of cardiac arrest to return to full consciousness is about two to three minutes elective ventilation may prove unnecessary. Unfortunately this is rare and is likely to occur only when the patient is already under intensive care. On a hospital ward, although the arrest is often witnessed, it may be many minutes before definitive treatment can be started. These patients will invariably need transfer to an intensive care unit for further assessment, monitoring, and treatment.

Accident and emergency departments receive patients who have had unwitnessed arrests. In these patients special attention must be given to cerebral resuscitation. All doctors who resuscitate patients must be aware of the consequences when resuscitation is incomplete and brain damage occurs. Nevertheless, more brains are damaged by inadequate than by inappropriate resuscitation. Experienced senior doctors must be involved early in the management of cardiac arrest, ideally from the start.

When the heart stops the brain may be damaged both by the initial ischaemia and by failure of adequate reperfusion. The latter is ultimately the most damaging. The brain may survive a period of hypoxia if cerebral flow is maintained. When cerebral blood flow ceases the electroencephalogram is flat within 10 seconds and cerebral glucose used up within one minute. Neuronal activity may, however, continue for up to an hour. Unfortunately progressive deterioration of the brain cannot be reversed or halted after about three minutes. A carotid pulse may be restored but the myriad of tiny cerebral vessels cannot be reperfused. Factors implicated are thought to include the following.

Vasospasm—Movement of calcium ions is implicated in vasospasm, and calcium antagonists have improved cerebral survival in animals. The administration of calcium during cardiac arrest must therefore be questioned and can be endorsed only for electromechanical dissociation.

Cerebral oedema—Hypoxia leads to cerebral oedema and this is augmented by the high blood levels of carbon dioxide associated with apnoea. Administration of sodium bicarbonate may release yet more carbon dioxide and compound the problem. Hyperventilation and elective lowering of the Pco_2 may reduce cerebral oedema and obviate the need for bicarbonate.

Microthrombus formation and sludging—When cerebral flow ceases the smaller vessels silt up. Once formed these blockages cannot be removed.

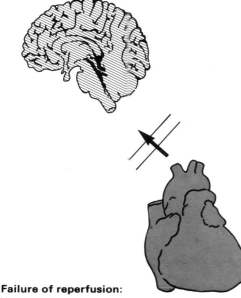

Failure of reperfusion:
Vasospasm
Cerebral oedema
Microthrombi and
 "sludging"

● Restore spontaneous cardiac output
● Control pH, blood gases
    and electrolytes
● Electively ventilate

Cerebral damage after cardiac arrest can be minimised by the following maneouvres.

Rapid return of spontaneous cardiac output—Cardiopulmonary resuscitation sometimes achieves no more than 5% of normal cerebral flow and minimal cerebral oxygenation. It does, however, prevent total cessation of cerebral blood flow.

Meticulous control of pH, blood gases, and electrolytes in the period immediately after the arrest. In most cases this can be achieved only by elective ventilation of a sedated paralysed patient in an intensive care unit.

Barbiturate coma may prevent the damaging effect of epileptic fits and protects against incomplete ischaemia, possibly by reducing cerebral activity. Barbiturates are mild calcium channel blockers and some are free radical scavengers. Their effectiveness is not proved or widely accepted.

Hypothermia reduces the activity of the brain but may itself induce cardiac arrest. It is technically difficult to achieve and is usually used when the patient is already hypothermic—for example, after near drowning.

Steroids—There is some evidence that steroids may modify the action of free radicals and so protect an ischaemic brain. They are valuable in controlling cerebral oedema associated with slow growing tumours but are of unproved value after an arrest.

Intracranial pressure monitoring—Cerebral perfusion pressure is the difference between mean arterial pressure and intracranial pressure. Careful monitoring of the intracranial pressure may help evaluate the efficacy of treatment.

Although spontaneous respiratory effort may return quite soon after a heart beat, it is rarely adequate and the gag reflex is usually impaired. A cuffed endotracheal tube will protect the airway and facilitate positive pressure ventilation. 100% Oxygen should be used in the early stages to ensure adequate oxygenation of poorly perfused areas. If the patient resists the endotracheal tube an immediate decision must be made about *elective ventilation*. This will allow hyperventilation to be used. A reduction of the Pco_2 to about 4 kPa (30 mm Hg) will reduce cerebral oedema, and control of ventilation will allow some correction of blood gas abnormalities and scrupulous maintenance of the Po_2.

A self expanding bag and valve are inadequate for more than a few minutes of resuscitation. They will allow carbon dioxide to build up, which can lead only to an increase in intracranial pressure and a deterioration in the acid base status. A mechanical ventilator must be used.

External chest compression may create a flail segment. This may be the result of rib fracture or, more commonly, of costochondral or sternal dislocation. Elective ventilation is mandatory in these circumstances. Do not wean a patient off a ventilator unless you know that the rib cage is intact.

Acid base balance

When an arrest was witnessed there is no need to administer sodium bicarbonate immediately. It need be given only when other methods have failed to reverse the acidosis. Even when the arrest was unwitnessed it is wise to administer bicarbonate only when there is a measured acidosis. External chest compression produces poor cerebral blood flow but even less peripheral circulation. There is little effective venous return, so lactic acid builds up but is not returned to the circulation until the heart is restarted. It is in the phase immediately after the arrest that serious acid base problems may occur, and continuous monitoring of the blood gases every 15 minutes, possibly for several hours, is essential. Sodium bicarbonate provides a large hyperosmolar sodium load to an extremely compromised circulation. It can produce a precipitous fall in the serum potassium concentration. It neutralises acid by the release of carbon dioxide, and a rise in the Pco_2 will lead to increased cerebral oedema. Carbon dioxide will move into the cerebrospinal fluid, making central

---

Immediately after restoration of cardiac rhythm complete this checklist

(1) With a laryngoscope ensure that the *endotracheal tube* is correctly placed in the trachea and not in the oesophagus

(2) Ensure that the patient is being adequately *ventilated* with *100% oxygen*. Listen with a stethoscope and confirm adequate and equal air entry. If you suspect *pneumothorax* insert a chest drain

(3) Estimate *arterial pH and gases*, preferably from an arterial sample, but use a central venous sample if necessary

(4) Estimate *serum potassium*

(5) Obtain a *chest radiograph*. An anteroposterior supine view is adequate

(6) Insert a *urinary catheter* and measure the urinary output

(7) Insert a *nasogastric tube* and aspirate the contents of the stomach

(8) Obtain a *12 lead electrocardiograph*

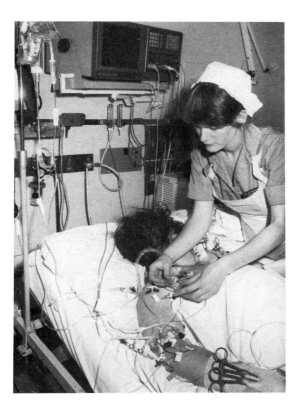

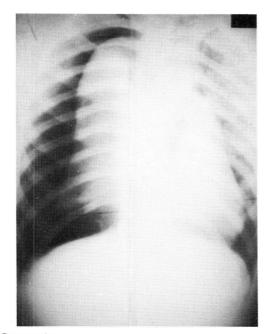
Pneumothorax

Lignocaine infusion

Add 2 g lignocaine (10 ml of 20% solution) to 500 ml 5% dextrose. Infuse at 5–15 drops a minute.

Caution

The pupillary responses of little value immediately after an arrest. Pupils dilate during cardiac arrest for several reasons. Concentrations of circulating endogenous catecholamines are very high immediately before and during an arrest and exogenous catecholamines are likely to have been given. Atropine may also have been administered. Ischaemia to the anterior chamber can dilate the pupils. Only when hypoxia has been corrected and the effects of drugs allowed to wear off can tests of brain stem function be employed. This may take several hours.

When feeling for carotid pulses, inserting a nasogastric tube, or replacing an endotracheal tube always watch the electrocardiographic monitor. Hypoxia augments many vagally mediated reflexes and stimulation of the carotid sinus or oropharynx under these circumstances may lead to marked reflex bradycardia and asystole.

monitoring of the pH by the brain extremely precarious once cardiac output has been restored. Blood gas and acid base abnormalities should initially be controlled by ventilation and the restoration of renal function. If these prove inadequate then small doses of bicarbonate can be given if blood gases are constantly monitored. Sodium bicarbonate should therefore never be given at the start of the procedure, must only be given to ventilated patients, and must be as a response to a known acid base abnormality.

Hypokalaemia may precipitate cardiac arrest, particularly in elderly patients taking digoxin and diuretics. Bicarbonate administration may further lower the serum potassium value. If the serum potassium concentration is very high, usually as the result of renal failure, then it can be lowered with glucose and insulin.

Each resuscitation attempt must be accompanied by a chest radiograph. Check the position of the central venous line and ensure that the endotracheal tube is not down a main bronchus. Pneumothorax may occur and is an important reversible cause of electromechanical dissociation. When electrical activity is recorded by the electrocardiogram but there is no cardiac output it is important to eliminate any other easily reversible condition. Cardiac tamponade may be diagnosed by an enlarged cardiac shadow and a raised central venous pressure. If in doubt obtain an echocardiogram.

Once a rhythm has been restored it is only of value if it produces an output. If you cannot feel a pulse continue external chest compression and treat the patient for electromechanical dissociation.

The haemodynamics of the period after an arrest are complex and must be measured if treatment is to be safe and effective. Palpation of the pulse and listening for Korotkoff sounds in the arm does not constitute measurement of the haemodynamics. A high systemic vascular resistance in a low flow state will prevent Korotkoff sounds being heard, despite a relatively high mean arterial pressure. Indwelling pulmonary and systemic arterial catheters must therefore be inserted to measure the true haemodynamic state before administering haemodynamically active drugs.

If a short period of hypertension ensues this is not harmful and may even be beneficial to the brain.

Consider a lignocaine infusion after ventricular fibrillation.

An adequate blood pressure will produce 40–50 ml of urine every hour. A urinary catheter may be necessary to monitor urine output.

Early attempts at mouth to mouth and bag and mask ventilation will have introduced air into the stomach. An initially misplaced endotracheal tube will do the same. Gastric distention provokes vomiting and is uncomfortable. It is usually necessary to insert a nasogastric tube.

The cause of the arrest and its effects on the heart may be shown by a 12 lead electrocardiogram. Any subsequent changes can be related to this early reading.

Conclusion

If patients are to be protected from the dangers inherent in our decision to resuscitate them we must accept that a commitment to treating cardiac arrest is a commitment to intensive postresuscitation care. The patient can be managed only in an intensive care unit and will need at least a short period of elective ventilation.

Newburg LA. Cerebral resuscitation: advances and controversies. *Ann Emerg Med* 1984;13:853–6.
White BC, Aust SD, Arfors KE, Aronson LD. Brain injury by ischaemic anoxia: hypotheses extension—a tale of ions? *Ann Emerg Med* 1984;13:862–7.
Niemann JT, Rosborough JP. Effects of acidaemic and sodium bicarbonate therapy in advanced cardiopulmonary resuscitation. *Ann Emerg Med* 1984;13:781–4.
Safar P. Recent advances in cardiocerebral resuscitation: a review. *Ann Emerg Med* 1984;13:856–2.
Redmond AD, Edwards JD. Haemodynamics during and after cardiac arrest. In: Vincent JL, ed. *Update in intensive care and emergency medicine.* Berlin: Springer, 1989:531–8.
Cohn, JN. Blood pressure measurement in shock. *JAMA* 1967,**199**:972–6.

TRAINING AND RETENTION OF SKILLS

GERALYN WYNNE

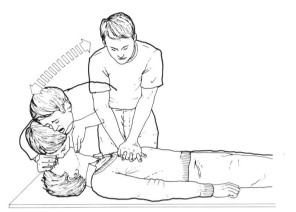

One person basic cardiopulmonary resuscitation

Better teaching of skills

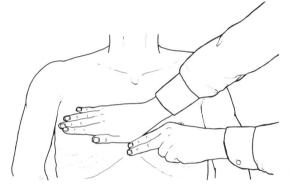

Landmarking

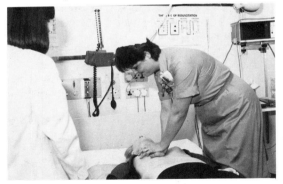

Cardiopulmonary resuscitation

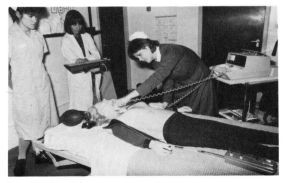

Training specialist nurses to defibrillate

Resuscitation training is essentially a practical skill and students need practical training to acquire it. Genuine life threatening situations rarely occur at a time or place where teaching is possible, so practical training has to be simulated. This has been made possible since 1960 by the development of various manikins and training aids.

In most hospitals teaching of resuscitation is haphazard, and medical and nursing students are perhaps taught only once during their courses. The teaching is usually left to a consultant or tutor interested in the subject, who is faced with a class of 20–40 students for one or two hours. There is probably no time during the session for students to practise what they are taught. Almost every hospital has a "training manikin", which is from time to time produced to entertain the class. How can these students be expected to perform resuscitation competently if they have never received adequate training?

The results of surveys of house officers' and trained nurses' inability to carry out cardiopulmonary resuscitation[1-4] suggest an urgent need for a review of resuscitation training. Formal training should begin in medical and nursing schools with no assumptions being made about previous knowledge. In 1987 The Royal College of Physicians published *Resuscitation from cardiopulmonary arrest: training and organisation*, which suggests that resuscitation skills may be considered at three levels:

(1) *Basic life support*—the combination of expired air resuscitation and external chest compressions. This should be taught to all unqualified nurses, physiotherapists, radiographers, preclinical students, and other staff who are in contract with patients and the public.

(2) *Basic life support with adjuncts*

(a) Basic life support with airway adjuncts should be taught to qualified nursing staff, basic trained ambulance staff, clinical medical students and general practitioners.

(b) Basic life support with airway adjuncts and defibrillation should be taught to all hospital medical staff, including house staff and all locum hospital doctors, specially trained nursing staff working in hospital areas such as the coronary care unit, intensive treatment unit, and accident and emergency department, and ambulance staff, and offered to general practitioners.

(3) *Advanced life support*—Every resuscitation team should be competent in eight areas of life support.

(a) Ability to perform basic life support
(b) Knowledge of specialist equipment
(c) Recognition of the mechanism of cardiac arrest
(d) Ability to treat life threatening cardiac arrhythmias and some other forms of cardiopulmonary arrest
(e) Ability to insert an intravenous line
(f) Techniques of mechanical ventilation
(g) Drugs and their dosage
(h) Recognition of the end points of resuscitation.

Revision courses for qualified doctors should be provided not just to instruct, but also to test skills. At present there is no recognised national training programme for basic or advanced life support in medical and nursing schools, though the Resuscitation Council (UK) has issued guidelines on basic and advanced life support, which are now being used in many centres.

Retaining skills

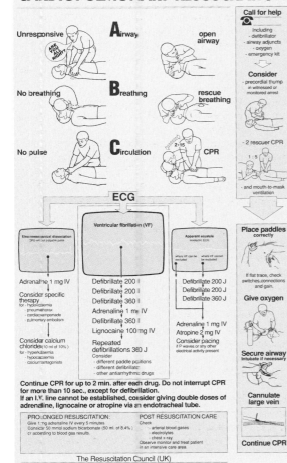

Since the development of the original resuscitation standards in 1974[5] in the USA investigators have concerned themselves with the question of how students attain and retain their skills. Particular interest has focused on how skills deteriorate over time.

Performance deteriorates over all intervals of time tested.[6] This is true even six weeks after training, and severe loss of skills occurs after about 12 months, when typically 20% or fewer trainees can perform basic life support proficiently. Individual differences in retention are found but are not related to differences in the sex or weight of the trainees. Decline in resuscitation skills is greater than for other first aid skills such as traction, splinting, or bandaging. The underlying theme is clear: skills that are not regularly practised are not retained.

The standards and guidelines for basic life support may seem complex, with different techniques and rules to be applied to one or two rescuers. Simplifying compression rates and compression: ventilation ratios for adult victims may maximise recall for the rescuer.

Acquiring and retaining cardiopulmonary resuscitation skills may also depend on the course content and time devoted to manikin practice.[7] When the American Heart Association standards are used as an evaluative tool the four hour teaching programme for one and two rescuer cardiopulmonary resuscitation and airway obstruction is associated with poor performance skills. Trainees who complete eight hours of instruction show less deterioration in skill than those who complete the usual four hour course. Although the two groups were not comparable in course content, trainees from the long course had significantly higher psychomotor performance scores, yet after one year even their standards were below those of the American Heart Association.

Several studies have concentrated on mastering the performance of basic resuscitation. For example, Canadian policemen were trained in one rescuer resuscitation only, and the length of the course was eight hours. At the end of the course they were tested and allowed three attempts, with remedial training, until they could master its performance. They were tested for retention of skills at 12–18 months, and no decrements were found in their ventilations or compressions.[8]

Do individuals who perform "poorly" in retention studies lack the ability to provide effective cardiopulmonary resuscitation in a real case? In one study poor technique was related to a poor outcome for the victim. Others, however, have failed to identify a relation between technique and the victim's survival.

Many cardiopulmonary resuscitation programmes in the USA do not give trainees the opportunity to attain the level of performance outlined by the American Heart Association. If trainees fail initially to achieve established cardiopulmonary resuscitation skills retention will certainly be poorer.

One British study evaluated 124 occupational first aiders who were tested on their ability to carry out cardiopulmonary resuscitation at varying times up to three years after training. Expert assessment of printouts from a recording manikin indicated that only 12% of those tested would have been capable of carrying out effective cardiopulmonary resuscitation. The same printouts also showed that there was a rapid and linear decay in resuscitation skills over time, with fewer than 20% of the subjects achieving a score of 75% on performance only six months after training. Variables such as age, sex, height, weight, and practice on a manikin did not influence performance.[9]

One reason for poor performance is rescuers' reluctance to perform expired air resuscitation. A survey of user acceptance of techniques of ventilation was carried out on 70 medical and nursing staff. Performance of these techniques—mouth to mouth, mouth to mask, bag valve mask, and oxygen powered resuscitator (Robertshaw)—was then measured in random order with a Wright's respirometer, before and after instruction, on a recording manikin in 35 subjects. Sixty four of the staff were not prepared to ventilate "dirty patients" (those who had vomited, had dirty sputum, or were infected) using mouth to

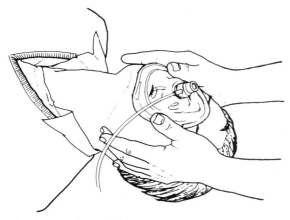

Mouth to mask ventilation

mouth resuscitation and 27 would not use mouth to mask ventilation.[10] Oral adjuncts need to be introduced to overcome user objections to "dirty patients"—for example, the pocket face mask, which can be used for mouth to face mask ventilation.[11]

One study tested the hypothesis that exposure to posters containing essential information on cardiopulmonary resuscitation displayed on lavatory walls improves theoretical knowledge and the performance of cardiopulmonary resuscitation. There was a significant increase in both knowledge and performance of cardiopulmonary resuscitation after exposure to posters.[12] This technique is inexpensive and simple and warrants more widespread use as a means of maintaining knowlege and proficiency in cardiopulmonary resuscitation.

Advanced life support

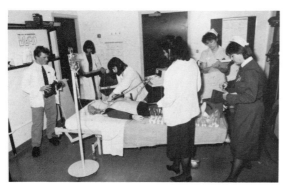

Equipment for simulated cardiac arrest
Manikin with a defibrillation torso
Electrocardiogram simulator
Airway adjuncts
Airway management trainer (optional)
Cardiac arrest trolley fully equipped with a defibrillator
Oxygen suction
Drugs

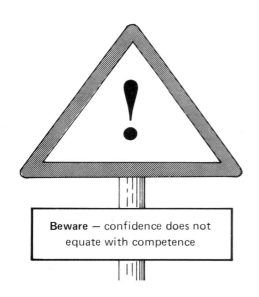

Simulated cardiac arrest

Beware — confidence does not equate with competence

The purpose of the advanced cardiac life support programme is to provide doctors, nurses, medical students, paramedics, and other allied health personnel with enough knowledge and practical skills to treat patients with cardiopulmonary arrest in real life. Kaye devised the megacode, designed to simulate an actual cardiac arrest, in which the students are offered the opportunity to integrate the knowledge and skills acquired in recognising arrhythmias, applying defibrillating electrodes on the arrhythmia manikin, practising intravenous cannulation, endotracheal intubation, airway management, and drug treatment to learn to act in a coordinated fashion as members of a resuscitation team.[13] Simulated cardiac arrests should be included in basic and advanced resuscitation training courses.

American studies have found that graduate and trained nurses, when questioned on orientation courses for newly qualified nurses, expressed feelings of being ineffective and insufficiently prepared to cope when faced with a real life cardiac arrest. Within the nursing programme they had completed basic life support training and had been orientated to resuscitation policies, procedures, and equipment in the hospital.[14] The problem was overcome by the use of simulated cardiac arrests. This gave the nurses the opportunity to practise their skills and to learn to work together in a coordinated fashion as members of a team. There is a need for tutorials to review the simulated cardiac arrest, which can be achieved by instructor feedback of performance and video recording. Unscheduled simulated cardiac arrests can be used to monitor the quality of resuscitation in hospital. These usually show unsuspected deficiencies in knowledge about cardiac arrests.[15]

A study performed to assess competence in advanced cardiac life support skills found that reinforcing and continuing medical education may enhance the retention of knowledge, but does not maintain motor skills.[16] Yearly recertification in advanced cardiac life support skills should be considered, and frequent simulated practice sessions should be encouraged for doctors and nurses.

One factor that may affect the acquisition of basic and advanced resuscitation skills is that when questioned 78% of medical students and residents felt confident of their ability to perform basic resuscitation, but only 2·9% did it correctly. Trained nurses at sister or charge nurse level felt significantly more confident than staff nurses at performing basic resuscitation, but were no more competent. This large discrepancy between imagined and actual ability will probably result in these people being unlikely to feel a need for additional training.

Experience and the number of arrests attended does not improve competency at basic resuscitation, although doctors and nurses are confident that they can perform the skills.

Medical student training

Preclinical

First year   St John first aid and resuscitation course in first term of preclinical year

Tested and given a certificate

Second year

Clinical

Third year
(1) Introductory two hour lecture
(2) Practical training in groups of 10 for one hour—basic life support, 1 or 2 rescuers

Anaesthetic module (two weeks)

Training for 1½ hours on:
(1) Revision basic life support, 1 or 2 rescuers
(2) Airway adjuncts, ventilation, oxygen cylinders
(3) Intubation tape slide presentation
Practical intubation on airway
Management trainers before supervision in theatre by anaesthetists
(4) Intravenous cannulation theatres

Tested in second week on:
(1) One rescuer resuscitation
(2) Airway adjuncts

Cardiothoracic module (six weeks)

Six one hour sessions on:
(1) Basic life support revision and airway adjuncts
Simulated basic life support situations
(2) Arrhythmias, basic electrocardiograms, identifying ventricular fibrillation, ventricular tachycardia, asystole, electromechanical dissociation, and bradycardia
(3) Management and drug dosage for ventricular fibrillation, ventricular tachycardia, asystole, electromechanical dissociation, and bradycardia
(4) Principles of defibrillation and defibrillators, practical training on arrhythmia manikin
(5) Postresuscitation care and role of team leader
(6) Simulated cardiac arrests

Fourth year

Fifth year
Two hour revision lecture on resuscitation.

Resuscitation test on:
(1) Basic life support
(2) Managing the airway
(3) Leadership skills, managing ventricular fibrillation

Resuscitation test part of final MB examination

The two schedules show the resuscitation training programmes currently followed by medical students at the Royal Free Hospital School of Medicine and to learner nurses at the Royal Free Hospital School of Nursing.

Teaching methods that can be used for basic life support and advanced cardiac life support training are as follows:

Verbal instruction—Clarity, accuracy, and repetition are necessary.

Visualisation—Techniques and procedures can be visualised in the form of demonstrations, blackboard pictures, charts, projected slides, films, and videos.

Practice is the most important aspect of cardiopulmonary resuscitation training. Training manikins must be used for practising lung ventilations and chest compressions. These should be as realistic as possible, to enhance motivation and physiologically correct learning. Each student should have enough time for manikin practice to reach perfection in performance. To achieve this lecturing should be kept to a minimum and student groups should be small. There should be no more than four to six students per manikin. Supervised practice allows guidance and evaluation by the instructor. The students should be tested before and after practice. They can be evaluated by printout records of their performance, which provide the evaluator with exact objective data, or by automatic guidance such as light signals, dials, printouts, etc.

Self training systems have many advantages over traditional lectures and manikin practice supervised by an instructor. People learn at different rates, so training programmes should allow for individualised learning. Self training systems should encourage students to acquire knowledge from illustrated texts, tape recorded lectures, or both. These systems guide skill practice on manikins through demonstration of pictures, coaching by audiotaped narration, or the text of manuals.

Learner nurse training for part I of the general register

(all training sessions two hours with six students to one manikin)

Foundation unit

Basic life support
(1) How to recognise a cardiopulmonary arrest
(2) Call for help—emergency bell or number
(3) Location of airway adjuncts
(4) Hands on practice (on the manikin) of basic life support and the use of airway adjuncts

Medicine 1 (week 17)
(1) Revision of basic life support and the use of airway adjuncts
(2) Hands on practice on the manikin

Introduction to medicine 2 (week 54)
(1) Revision of previous learning
(2) Introduction to the cardiac arrest trolley
(3) Role of the nurse in a cardiac arrest
(4) Practical skill session, how to help with intubation, use prepacked syringes, etc
(5) Discussion about participation in managing cardiac arrests and role of the nurse

Introduction to theatres (week 74)
(1) Revision of skills necessary for managing patients in theatre and recovery

Paediatric module (week 96)
(1) Resuscitation of infants and children
(2) Hands on practice with Resusci baby and junior

Trauma (week 106)
(1) Revision of basic resuscitation skills
(2) Role of the nurse in a cardiac arrest in the accident and emergency department
(3) Recognising and managing life threatening arrhythmias

Management teaching (week 141)
(1) Practical basic resuscitation test (surprise)
(2) Revision of basic resuscitation skills
(3) Problem solving exercise—the role of the staff nurse in a cardiac arrest

Recommendations for improving the quality of cardiopulmonary resuscitation training

(1) Practical training on a manikin is better than either demonstration only or passive learning.

(2) Feedback is essential, especially via a recording and monitoring manikin and video recording. The students should be tested before and after training.

(3) Practice after initial training improves cardiopulmonary resuscitation performance.

(4) Refresher training is important; even a brief review of training material can have a measurable effect.

(5) Periodic refresher training is essential if the skill is to be retained and should take place probably within a year of training.

(6) Guidelines for training should be as uniform as possible and at least similar throughout the world.

(7) Schools should play a part in disseminating knowledge about first aid and cardiopulmonary resuscitation and in teaching proficiency to the public at large. School age is excellent for learning these relatively simple psychomotor skills and the necessary knowledge. Teaching school children allows for yearly retraining.

(8) Ideally every hospital should have a resuscitation training room equipped with all the appropriate training aids for basic and advanced life support. Trainees shuld be encouraged to visit the room in small groups to use the equipment at their own pace and under the direction and supervision of a resuscitation training officer.

(9) A designated resuscitation training officer is vital for coordinating and implementing resuscitation training programmes within a hospital if standards and skills are to be maintained.

Adequate training in resuscitation should provide the knowledge, skills, reassurance, and motivation necessary for achieving a competent performance in real life.

1 Casey WF. CPR—a survey of standards among junior hospital doctors. *J R Soc Med* 1984; 77: 921–3.
2 Lowenstein SR. CPR by medical and surgical house officers. Lancet 1981; ii: 679–81.
3 Skinner D. CPR skills of preregistration house officers. *Br Med J* 1985; 290: 1549–50.
4 Wynne GA. Inability of trained nurse to perform basic life support. *Br Med J* 1987; 294: 1198–9.
5 American Heart Association. Standards and guidelines for cardiopulmonary resuscitation and emergency cardiac care. *JAMA* 1974; 227: 833–68.
6 Latman NS, Wooley K. Knowledge and skill retention of emergency care attendants EMT As and EMT Ps. *Ann Emerg Med* 1981; 9: 182–3.
7 Gombeski WR Jr, Effron DM, Ramirez AG, Moore TJ. Impact on retention: comparison of two CPR training programs. *Am J Public Health* 1982; 72: 849–52.
8 Tweed WA, Wilson E, Isfeld B. Retention of cardiopulmonary resuscitation skills after initial overtraining. *Crit Care Med* 1980; 8: 651–3.
9 McKenna SP, Glendon AI. Occupational first aid training. Decay in CPR skills. *Journal of Occupational Psychology* 1985; 58: 109–17.
10 Lawrence PJ, Sivaneswaran N. Ventilation during CPR—which method? *Anaesth Intensive Care* 1985; 13: 201.
11 Seidelin PH, Stolarek IH, Littlewood DG. Comparison of six methods of emergency ventilation. *Lancet* 1986; ii:1274.
12 Grogono AW, Jastremski MS, Johnson MM, Russell RF. Educational graffiti. Better use of the lavatory wall. *Lancet* 1982; i 1175–6.
13 Kaye W, Linhares KC, Breault RV, Norris PA, Stamoulis CC, Khan AH. The mega code for training the advanced cardiac life support team. *Heart Lung* 1981; 10: 860–5.
14 Matson C, Spears B. Simulated cardiopulmonary arrest. A planned learning experience. *Focus on Critical Care* 1985; 12: 19–21.
15 Sullivan MJJ, Guyatt GH. Simulated cardiac arrests for monitoring the quality of in hospital resuscitation. *Lancet* 1986; ii: 618–620.
16 Stross JK. Maintaining competency in ACLS skills. *JAMA* 1983; 249: 3339–41.
17 Royal College of Physicians. Resuscitation from cardiopulmonary arrest training and organisation. *J R Coll Physicians Lon* 1987; 21: 1–8.

TRAINING MANIKINS

ROBERT S SIMONS, ANNE R CHAMNEY

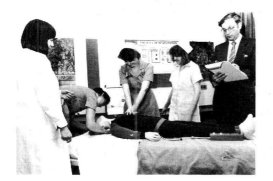

Training in cardiopulmonary resuscitation embodies theoretical and practical skills. For theoretical teaching audiovisual material is available from national organisations and commercial sources. Practical training requires manikins, and teachers of cardiopulmonary resuscitation need to be aware of the requirements of their target audience and the facilities available in different models.

Although more detailed reviews of training manikins for cardiopulmonary resuscitation are available,[1][2] this chapter examines current models from three manufacturers whose products are readily available in the UK, and lists the addresses of some other manufacturers.

Training requirements

Skill expectation

Basic life support
Airway control (±simple airways)
Mouth clearance, management of choking
Expired air resuscitation (±adjuncts)
Pulse detection
External cardiac compression
Posture including recovery position
Control of haemorrhage and fractures
Paediatric resuscitation

Advanced cardiac life support
Resuscitation airways
Suction equipment
Manual resuscitators (±mechanical devices)
Endotracheal intubation
ECG diagnosis
Defibrillation and cardioversion
Intravenous access and drug therapy
Neonatal resuscitation
Circulation support (MAST garments, etc)

Citizen cardiopulmonary resuscitation programmes have quite different requirements from those for professional hospital staff.[3] A guide to skill expectation is given in the box, although the division between basic and advanced cardiopulmonary resuscitation is not absolute. The American Heart Association endorses basic life support without airway or ventilatory devices,[4] but training for healthcare workers should include the use of simple airway adjuncts.

Manikin selection

Manikin selection

Audience—size, standard, training frequency
Realistic anatomy—landmarks and appearance
Multiple and concurrent task capability
Response to resuscitation manoeuvres
Visible display of performance
Permanent record facility
Objective scoring capability
Safety (cross infection and electrical risks, etc)
Durability
Ease of maintenance and repair
Portability
Power requirements
Cost

When choosing a manikin, lifelike anatomical appearance and realistic function are essential. Other factors as outlined alongside should also be considered. In addition staff must be available for teaching students and maintaining equipment, and space must be provided for training and storage. Manikins should be easy to clean, and the skin should not stain from contact with lipstick, ball point, or marker pens or discolour after extensive handling. Moreover the skin should be strengthened against splitting at vulnerable junctions, such as the corners of the mouth or eyes. Components liable to wear and tear, such as the face, skin, and chest piece, should if possible be easy to replace. Stranded hair may look realistic but is difficult to clean and constitutes an unwarranted risk of infection.

To minimise the risk of cross infection using manikins, the numbers of students for each manikin should be kept small and attention to hygiene should be careful. Manikins should be disinfected during and after each training session.[5] Face shields and other disposables should be changed between students, and the manikin's face should be cleaned with 70% alcohol or 500 ppm chlorine (20 ml bleach/litre water), allowing 30 seconds contact time. Between classes the manikin should be disassembled, washed with soapy water, and the surfaces wetted for 10 minutes with fresh dilute bleach solution as above, then rinsed and dried.

New practices in cardiopulmonary resuscitation may not be demonstrable on models designed several years ago—for example, treatment of choking by abdominal thrust, use of the recovery position, management of trauma and haemorrhage, and the use of resuscitation airway adjuncts.

Basic life support

Ambu		
ABC manikin (torso),	£	197
Ambu Man (basic torso)	£	540
(+instruments)	£	600
(+computer interface)	£	692
(+full body)	add £	130
Laerdal		
Anatomic Anne (torso)	£	350
Resusci Anne (torso)	£	270–410
Resusci Anne (full size)	£	525
Recording Resusci Anne	£	850
Resusci Baby	£	200–320
Resusci Junior	£	385
Skillmeter Resusci Anne	£	1075
printer	+ £	220

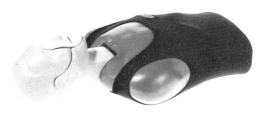

Ambu ABC

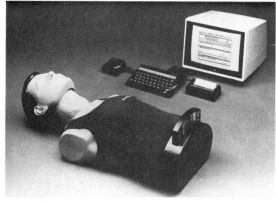

Ambu Man

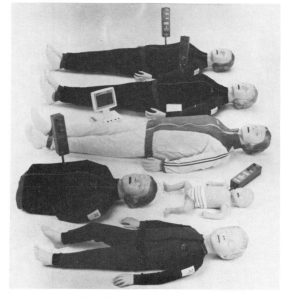

Laerdal's manikins (from above): Resusci Anne,
Recording Resusci Anne, Skillmeter Resusci Anne,
Resusci Anne torso, Resusci Baby, and Resusci Junior

Although not as realistic, torso models are more portable than full size manikins.

Ambu ABC is a simple model primarily designed for rescue breathing only.

Ambu Man is a new manikin that supersedes the Ambu-S CPR simulator. It has the same method of displacing expired air into a disposable plastic bag in the head shell as used in previous models. The head movements and general appearance of the manikin have been considerably improved, and limbs can be added. An inflatable stomach and supervisor-controlled carotid pulse are included. A desirable option is the plug-in monitoring unit that displays tidal volume and cardiac compression responses and indicates wrong hand position and stomach inflation. An interface to a Spectrum computer and printer can provide a graphic or text display of several variables recorded for 1, 5, or 10 minutes with an analysis of the candidate's performance. The criteria are strict and based on American Heart Association guidelines.

The Laerdal Resusci manikins include a range of torso and full bodied models, most of which can be connected to an indicator light box to show adequate ventilation, adequate compression, or wrong hand position.

Recording Resusci Anne also has a metronome and a battery operated, pressure sensitive, paper strip writer that provides a permanent record of the rescuer's attempts at ventilation and cardiac compression.

Resusci Junior simulates a 5 year old child for practising cardiopulmonary resuscitation and water rescue (floating or submerged). Understandably, it lacks electrical indicators. It is particularly suitable for teaching lifesavers, playschool nurses, and children.

Resusci Baby is a very realistic model for teaching infant resuscitation.

Skillmeter Resusci Anne has recently been added and features a computerised monitor with liquid crystal display screen. Sensors in the manikin respond to the rescuer's attempts at shaking, carotid palpation, and airway opening. Other sensors monitor ventilation and compression, and rates, ratios, and performance of the resuscitation manoeuvres can be calculated and displayed. A paper strip recorder listing correct and incorrect performance is available.

Some models can also be used for teaching further skills, such as basic nursing care (Adam Rouilly, CLA, Gaumard) and first aid management of haemorrhage and fractures (Alderson, San Arena) Many of these manikins may be used to test skills in rescue and transportation under a wide range of conditions. Other baby manikins, ranging from the premature baby to infant models are also available (Simulaids).

Airway control, management of choking, and recovery position

The facility to tilt the neck or lift the jaw, or both, is a feature of most manikins, though the necks of some cannot be rotated. Many earlier manikins required excessive neck extension to achieve a patent airway, which would be hazardous if performed on real casualties with associated neck injuries. In Ambu Man, Resusci Junior, and Skillmeter Resusci Anne stomach inflation will occur if expired air resuscitation is attempted while the airway is obstructed.

Earlier manikins for basic life support generally had small mouths with rudimentary oral cavities and tongues, which made the practice of mouth sweeps and inserting resuscitation airways virtually impossible. This problem has been rectified in newer models such as Ambu Man and Skillmeter Resusci Anne.

Back blows and abdominal thrusts can only be practiced on appropriately designed manikins (Simulaids). Adoption of the recovery position is impracticable for manikins lacking jointed body and limbs, though the posture can be shown on volunteers. Resusci Junior is notably lifelike in this respect.

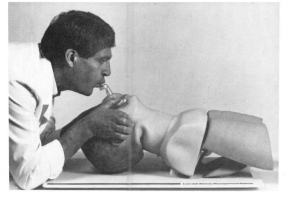

Mouth to face mask on a manikin

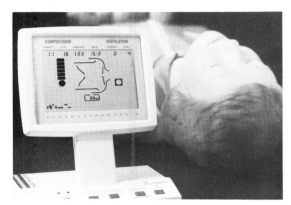

Skillmeter Resusci Anne

Rescue breathing

Considerations for expired air resuscitation include realistic compliance and resistance, a suitable display of ventilatory performance, and an effective means of avoiding cross infection. Ambu relies on a clean mouthpiece and a disposable bag insert in the manikin's head for each rescuer. Laerdal offers disposable face shields for each rescuer and replaceable lower airways and lung bags, and incorporate a valve to duct expired gases to the side of the manikin during expiration.

Mouth to nose ventilation is difficult to perform on these manikins because they have small noses, which are too soft, lack septa, and have inadequate nostrils. The noses were designed simply to be pinched closed during resuscitation, and access for nasal airways and catheters is impossible. Expired air resuscitation by facemask depends on the quality of seal between mask and face and is best performed using a mask with an inflatable cuff. Bag and mask ventilation requires a very firm one handed grip, and gas leaks readily occur, whereas mouth to mask ventilation using a two handed grip is easy to manage even by inexperienced people.

Cardiac compression

Essential requirements for cardiac compression include appropriate chest wall compliance and recoil and a suitable display of circulatory performance, including adequate depth of compression and wrong hand position. The latter feature is still not standardised between models.

Carotid pulses can be palpated on several adult manikins. These are generally not activated by rescuer compression but require the supervisor to operate a squeeze bulb to simulate the pulse. In infant models the brachial pulse is palpable in accordance with current practices.

Advanced cardiac life support

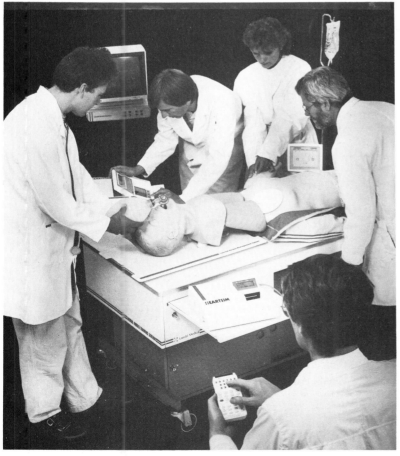

Megacode training in progress

The development of manikins for advanced resuscitation has proceeded piecemeal. No single manikin presently tests all the skills required for an interactive or team approach. One way of overcoming this problem is to group various manikins in a teaching room,[6] while Kaye has used elements of several models to construct a manikin for teaching his megacode scheme.[7]

Laerdal	
Arrhythmia Anne 2000 (complete)	£3200
Heartsim 2000 rhythm simulator	£1550
Skillmeter Arrhythmia Anne	£1450
Intubation	
Ambu airway intubation trainer	£410
Laerdal airway management trainer	£575
Laerdal infant intubation model	£140

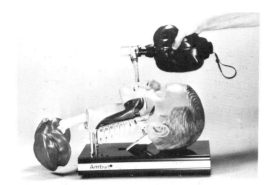

Adult intubation trainer (Ambu)

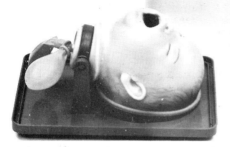

Infant intubation trainer (Laerdal)

Tracheal intubation

Tracheal intubation manikins require an extended head, a large open mouth, and accurate pharyngolaryngeal anatomy. Various features offered on the UK models include: postuable head and neck, the use of resuscitation airways, the ability to practise oropharyngeal suction, facilities for oral and nasal intubation, an audible alarm for excessive jaw force, variable laryngeal position, and changeable dental configurations. There is also an infant version.

Ambu's model has a cut away section of the left face and neck to improve visualisation of technique, whereas Laercal and Vitalograph provide a second laryngeal assembly alongside the head for atraumatic practice before intubating the manikin. A facility for bronchoscopy is offered as an optional extra on models by Laerdal and CLA.

Careful choice of a robust trainer is recommenced, and lubricant spray should always be used. Damage to mouth, tongue, and larynx is common, so it is desirable to be able to repair the trainer in house.

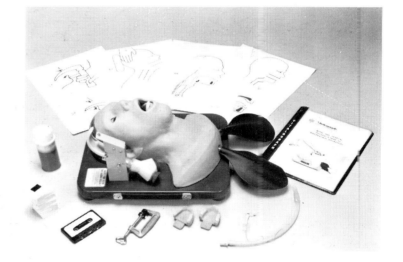

RFH intubation trainer (Vitalograph)

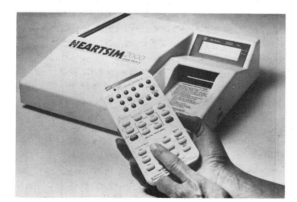

Adult airway management trainer (Laerdal)

Heartsim 2000 rhythm simulator (Laerdal)

Cardiac rhythm and defibrillation

Real time rhythm changes on an oscilloscope are more realistic than leisurely inspection of static rhythm strips. Simulators have been available for years using magnetic tape cartridges, cassettes, or solid state filter networks, but microprocessor technology offers extended capabilities. Laerdal's new Heartsim 2000 replaces Arrhythmia Anne IV and connects to Recording or Skillmeter Resusci Anne using a special torso skin with paddle electrode and attenuator box. It offers a wide range of arrhythmia patterns and includes a self instruct mode. Training in defibrillation techniques using standard defibrillators is a feature of the system. An optional monitor interface to a TV or video monitor is available and different plug-in program modules show a range of respiratory and haemodynamic electrocardiogram wave forms.

It should be remembered that energies of 50–400 J are associated with potentially lethal voltages of 2·5–7 kV.

Intravenous access

Laerdal's infusion arm (£160) allows percutaneous venepuncture to be practised, although the simulation of tactile sense and elasticity is disappointing. Several other manufacturers produce similar models, and a particularly realistic torso model for central venous cannulation of internal jugular and subclavian veins is available (Nasco).

Further considerations

UK distributors

Ambu International UK Ltd, Charlton Rd,
Midsomer Norton, Bath BA3 4DR
(0761 416868)

Laerdal Medical Ltd, Goodmead Rd,
Orpington, Kent BR6 0HX (0689 76634)

Vitalograph Ltd, Maids Moreton House,
Buckingham MK18 1SW (0280 813691)

Other distributors

Actronics, 810 River Avenue, Pittsburgh, PA
15212, USA

Adam Rouilly (London) Ltd, Crown Quay
Lane, Sittingbourne, Kent ME10 3JG

Alderson Research Labs Inc, 390 Ludlow St,
PO Box 1271, Stanford, CT 06904, USA

Brunswick Manufacturing Co Inc, 90 Myrtle
St, North Quincy, MA, USA

P Burtscher (San Arena), Buhlwiesenstrasse
25, CH 8600 Dubendorf, Switzerland

CLA, Coburger Lehrmittelanstalt, Postfach
650, 8630 Coburg, West Germany

Gaumard Scientific Co Inc, PO Box 140098,
Coral Gables, Florida 33114–0098, USA

Koken Co Ltd (Koken Resim), 5–18
Shimoochiai, 3 Chome, Shinjuku-Ku, Tokyo
161, Japan

NASCO, 901 Janesville Ave, Fort Atkinson,
Wisconsin 53538, USA

Simulaids Inc, PO Box 807, 271 Tinker Street,
Woodstock, NY 12498, USA

1 Emergency Care Research Institute. Training manikins, CPR. *Health Devices* 1981;10:227–53.
2 Simons RS. Training aids and models. In: PJF Baskett, ed. *Cardiopulmonary resuscitation.* Amsterdam: Elsevier Biomedical Press, 1989; Ch 16:347–83.
3 Safar P, Bircher NG. Teaching of first aid and resuscitation. In: *Cardiopulmonary cerebral resuscitation.* 3rd ed. Philadelphia: WB Saunders, 1981: 339–59. (Available from Laerdal.)
4 American Heart Association. Standards and guidelines for cardiopulmonary resuscitation and emergency cardiac care. *JAMA* 1986;255:2841–30–4.
5 Committee for Evaluation of Sanitary Practices in CPR Training. Recommendations for decontaminating manikins used in cardiopulmonary resuscitation training. *Resp Care* 1984; 29:1250–2.
6 Baskett PJF, Lawler PGP, Hudson RBS, Makepeace APW, Cooper C. A resuscitation teaching room in a district general hospital. *Br Med J* 1976;i:568–71.
7 Kaye W, Linhares KC, Breault RV, Norris PA, Stamoulis CC, Khan AH. The *Mega-Code* for training the advanced cardiac life support team. *Heart Lung* 1981;10:860–5.
8 Kaye W, Mancini ME. Evaluation with the *Mega-Code* of the performance of the advanced cardiac life support team. *Crit Care Med* 1986;14:99–102.
9 Hon DF. Interactive training in cardiopulmonary resuscitation. *Byte* 1982;7(No 6):108–38
10 Simons RS. Computerised training manikin for advanced cardiac life support. *Care of the Critically Ill* 1986;2:205–7.
11 Abrahamson S, Wallace P. Using computer controlled interactive manikins in medical education. *Medical Teacher* 1980; 2:25–31.

Display of performance—During cardiopulmonary resuscitation the trainee, supervisor, and audience need clear, concise, and objective indications of performance. It is important to identify inadequate, correct, or excessive force. Lights or buzzers can provide only a "yes/no" indication, whereas analogue meters display a quantitative value. The ability to make a permanent record is particularly useful for group teaching, retrospective analysis, and examination.

Evaluation of progress in resuscitation—The current UK manikins are not capable of "spontaneous" responses, although most feature a carotid pulse that can be controlled by the supervisor.

There is a need for automated respiratory and circulatory activity and for clinical indicators such as "blood oxygenation", "cerebral responsiveness", and "pupil response", which would enable the trainee to assess progress in resuscitation.

Concurrent task performance/team interaction—Successful resuscitation requires the integration of multiple tasks, whether performed by a sole rescuer or by a team. Testing of team skills is limited only by the ingenuity of the instructor or physical limitation such as power supply. For testing advanced cardiopulmonary skills Kaye uses a "megacode" to test the team leader and members in a scenario of cardiorespiratory problems requiring appropriate clinical management.[8]

Recommendations—Hospitals must be responsible for maintaining resuscitation standards among medical, nursing, and auxiliary staff. A district general hospital needs at least two adult manikins, and a baby or child manikin is essential for training in paediatric resuscitation.

For advanced cardiopulmonary resuscitation doctors and nurses in specialised units require access to adult and neonatal intubation trainers and an arrhythmia generator (with or without torso capability).

The burden of teaching has traditionally fallen on anaesthetists, cardiologists, and accident and emergency specialists. The tasks of organisation, training, and maintenance of equipment are time consuming if performed properly and merit the appointment of a designated resuscitation training officer, probably with a nursing or paramedical background. Such a person will unify and improve the quality of training and should be affordable within a district hospital's budget.

Future developments—The use of a microcomputer and video screen to measure performance and display results graphically is already feasible. There is increasing development of sophisticated simulators using computer technology (San Arena, Koken Resim) but these are too costly for most basic cardiopulmonary resuscitation schemes. Hon describes an ingenious computer operated manikin trainer linked to a video disc,[9] subsequently developed by Actronics. It requires no supervision and has obvious potential for mass training but is expensive and requires careful maintenance. The market for advanced cardiopulmonary resuscitation trainers is small but demanding and eager for new training techniques. A potential example of a computerised manikin has been described.[10]

In 1967 Sim I, costing some $100 000, was built as the ultimate in manikin technology.[11] The next few years will surely see the introduction of affordable and practical simulators at all levels of life support training.

RESUSCITATION IN PREGNANCY

G A D REES, B A WILLIS

Acute causes of 138 maternal deaths out of 209 deaths in pregnancy		
Cause		*No of deaths*
Haemorrhage	49	
Uteroplacental		24
Cerebrovascular		25
associated with:		
Pre-clampsia		6
Eclampsia		8
Non-obstetric		11
Embolism	41	
Pulmonary		25
Amniotic fluid		14
Air or gas		2
Cardiac	14	
Ischaemic heart disease		6
Eisenmenger's syndrome		4
Other		4
Anaesthesia	19	
Failed intubation		10
Pulmonary aspiration		5
Epidural analgesia		1
Other		3
Status epilepticus	7	
Unknown cause	8	

Cardiac arrest in late pregnancy occurs about once in 30 000 pregnancies,[1] and survival of such an event is exceptional.[2] The most recent report on maternal mortality shows that most maternal deaths are due to acute causes,[1] hence resuscitation skills are required of all staff directly or indirectly involved in obstetric care.

Factors peculiar to pregnancy that weight the balance against survival include anatomical considerations that may result in difficulty in maintaining a clear airway and intubating, pathological changes such as laryngeal oedema, and physiological factors such as increased oxygen consumption and an increased likelihood of pulmonary aspiration. However, the most important factor of all in the third trimester is inferior vena caval compression by the gravid uterus when the pregnant patient lies supine. This impairs venous return and withstands the most competent resuscitative efforts.

Anatomical features relevant to difficult intubation or ventilation

Difficult intubation:
- Full dentition
- Large breasts
- Oedema or obesity of neck
- Supraglottic oedema

Difficult external chest compression:
- Inferior vena caval compression by gravid uterus
- Flared ribcage
- Raised diaphragm

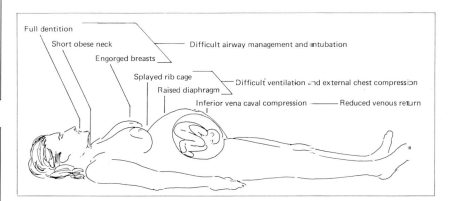

Supine pregnant patient

Physiological changes in late pregnancy relevant to cardiopulmonary resuscitation

Respiratory:
- Increased ventilation
- Increased oxygen demand
- Reduced chest compliance
- Reduced functional residual capacity

Cardiovascular:
- Increased cardiac output

Gastrointestinal:
- Incompetent gastro-oesophageal (cardiac) sphincter
- Increased intragastric pressure
- Increased risk of regurgitation

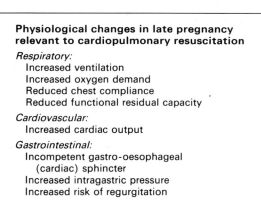

Speedy response is essential. Once a respiratory or cardiac arrest has been diagnosed, the patient must be positioned appropriately and basic life support started immediately. Basic life support must be continued while venous access is secured, any obvious causal factors such as hypovolaemia are corrected, and the equipment, drugs, and staff for advanced life support are assembled.

Basic life support

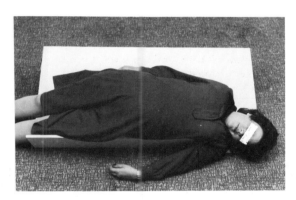

Cardiff resuscitation wedge

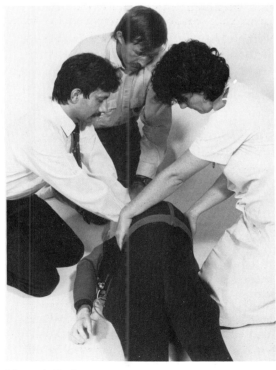

Manual displacement

Airway

A clear airway must be established quickly and maintained to resuscitate successfully any collapsed patient. Suction aspirating vomit, removing dentures or foreign bodies from the mouth, and inserting an airway improves airway patency and ventilation. These procedures should be performed with the patient inclined laterally or supine and with the uterus displaced (see below).

Breathing

In the absence of adequate respiration, intermittent positive pressure ventilation must be started once the airway has been cleared; mouth to mouth, mouth to nose, or mouth to airway ventilation should be continued until a bag and mask is available and the ventilation continued with 100% oxygen.

Ventilation of pregnant patients is made relatively difficult by their increased oxygen requirements and reduced chest compliance because of rib flaring and diaphragmatic splinting by the abdominal contents. Observing the rise and fall of the chest in such patients is also more difficult.

Because of the increased risk of regurgitation and pulmonary aspiration of gastric contents in late pregnancy, cricoid pressure should be applied until the airway is protected by endotracheal intubation with a cuffed tube.

Circulation

Circulatory arrest is diagnosed by the absence of palpable pulses in the large arteries (carotid or femoral). External chest compression at a rate of 60–80 compressions a minute must be started immediately, pausing briefly every five compressions for ventilation (one inflation of the lungs) if there are two resuscitators, or every 15 compressions for ventilation (two inflations) if there is a single resuscitator.

External chest compression of pregnant patients is rendered difficult by flared ribs, raised diaphragm, obesity, and breast hypertrophy. In the supine position an additional factor is inferior vena caval compression by the gravid uterus,[3] which impairs venous return and so reduces cardiac output. *All attempts at resuscitation will therefore be futile unless inferior vena caval compression is relieved.* This can be achieved either by placing the patient in an inclined lateral position using a wedge or by displacing the uterus from the great vessels manually.

The Cardiff resuscitation wedge

Effective forces for external chest compression can be generated with patients inclined at angles up to 30°,[4] but because of their anatomical changes pregnant patients tend to roll into a full lateral position when inclined laterally at angles of more than 30°, which makes external chest compression difficult. The Cardiff resuscitation wedge was designed based on these observations, and it was manufactured by the appropriate hospital department. To be portable but substantial enough to withstand resuscitative efforts the wedge is made from plywood and laminated for easy cleaning. The position of the patient permits good access by resuscitation and obstetric staff and enables the patient's head to be positioned by pillows for intubation and inserting a central line. In studies using a mannikin on the Cardiff resuscitation wedge, mouth to mouth ventilation and external chest compression were as effective in the laterally inclined position as in the supine.[4]

Manual displacement

If some form of resuscitation wedge is not available the patient should be placed supine on a hard surface to permit conventional basic life support and external chest compression in the usual way. An assistant must, however, move the uterus off the inferior vena cava by bimanually lifting it to the left and towards the patient's head to relieve inferior venal caval compression.

Despite the difficulties outlined above in performing basic life support in pregnant patients, basic life support must be regarded as the reflex response to cardiorespiratory arrest until equipment, staff, and drugs for advanced life support are available.

Advanced life support

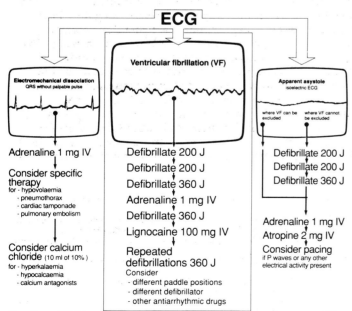

Ventilation

Intubation

Head and neck positions for ventilation and intubation

ECG

Electromechanical dissociation QRS without palpable pulse	Ventricular fibrillation (VF)	Apparent asystole isoelectric ECG
		where VF can be excluded / where VF cannot be excluded
Adrenaline 1 mg IV	Defibrillate 200 J	Defibrillate 200 J

Consider specific therapy
for - hypovolaemia
  - pneumothorax
  - cardiac tamponade
  - pulmonary embolism
	Defibrillate 200 J
	Defibrillate 360 J
	Adrenaline 1 mg IV
	Defibrillate 360 J
	Lignocaine 100 mg IV
		Defibrillate 200 J
		Defibrillate 360 J

		Adrenaline 1 mg IV Atropine 2 mg IV

Consider calcium chloride (10 ml of 10%)
for - hyperkalaemia
  - hypocalcaemia
  - calcium antagonists
	Repeated defibrillations 360 J
	Consider
	- different paddle positions
	- different defibrillator
	- other antiarrhythmic drugs
		Consider pacing
		if P waves or any other electrical activity present

Continue CPR for up to 2 min. after each drug. Do not interrupt CPR for more than 10 sec., except for defibrillation.
If an I.V. line cannot be established, consider giving double doses of adrenaline, lignocaine or atropine via an endotracheal tube.

PROLONGED RESUSCITATION:	POST RESUSCITATION CARE
Give 1 mg adrenaline IV every 5 minutes. Consider 50 mmol sodium bicarbonate (50 ml. of 8.4%) or according to blood gas results.	Check - arterial blood gases - electrolytes - chest x-ray Observe monitor and treat patient in an intensive care area.

Drugs and defibrillation

Intubation

The trachea should be intubated as soon as facilities and expertise are available. Pregnant patients may be difficult to intubate because of changes caused by pregnancy. In particular, a short obese neck and full breasts make inserting the laryngoscope into the mouth difficult. Using a laryngoscope with its blade mounted at more than 90° (Polio or adjustable blade) or demounting the blade from the handle during its insertion into the mouth can help.

Intubation usually follows a period of mask or mouth to mouth ventilation, which is best undertaken without pillows under the head and with the head and neck fully extended. The position for intubation, however, requires at least one pillow flexing the neck, with the head extended on the neck. The pillow removed to facilitate mask ventilation must therefore be kept at hand to position the head and neck for intubation.

Defibrillation and drugs

Defibrillation and drug administration to the pregnant patient during advanced life support should be in accordance with the revised recommendations of the Resuscitation Council (UK).[5]

Adrenaline (1 mg intravenously) is the first drug of choice after defibrillation; in addition to inotropic and chronotropic effects it has cerebral salvaging potential by maintaining cerebral circulation during prolonged resuscitation. Clinical evidence shows that external chest compression is ineffective when cardiac arrest is associated with sympathetic blockade (such as with epidural and spinal analgesia and anaesthesia) as peripheral blood flow is increased at the expense of vital organ perfusion.[6] Rapid administration of adrenaline is essential for its vasoconstrictive α agonist activity to increase venous return and cardiac output during external chest compression.

Intravenous administration of atropine (2 mg) to manage bradycardia and lignocaine (100 mg) to treat ventricular tachycardia and as prophylaxis against ventricular fibrillation also have a role in advanced life support.

Experimental evidence suggests that, should a cardiac arrest result from the cardiotoxic effects of inadvertant intravascular injection of the local anaesthetic agent, bupivicaine, the drug of choice other than adrenaline is bretylium tosylate (500 mg intravenously slowly), rather than lignocaine.[7]

Sodium bicarbonate (50 ml of 8.4%) should be given intravenously during prolonged resuscitation, preferably after arterial blood gas measurement of base deficit and after ventilation to normocapnia (4 kPa near term), to minimise respiratory acidosis.

Also in accordance with the revised recommendations of the Resuscitation Council (UK), the intravenous route is preferred for drug administration, and endotracheal administration should only be used if intravenous access is not available. The intracardiac administration of adrenaline is not recommended by the Council, and in pregnant patients anatomical changes make accurate placement of such injections unlikely.

Caesarean section

It is becoming appreciated that caesarean section is not merely a last ditch attempt to save the life of the fetus but plays an important part in the resuscitation of the mother. This is attested by many reports that describe successful resuscitation after prompt surgical intervention.[8-12] The probable mechanism for the favourable outcome is that inferior vena caval occlusion is relieved completely by emptying the uterus, whereas it is only relieved partially by using the lateral position.[13]

The speed of the surgical delivery is critical to the outcome for both arrested mother and fetus. In arrested non-pregnant adults irreversible brain damage from anoxia occurs within 3–4 minutes, but arrested pregnant patients become hypoxic more quickly.[14] Although there is evidence that fetuses are able to tolerate prolonged periods of hypoxia,[12, 15] neonatal outcome is optimised by immediate caesarean section.

If maternal cardiac arrest occurs in the labour ward, operating theatre, or casualty department, and basic and advanced life support are not successful within five minutes, the uterus should be emptied by surgical intervention. Cardiopulmonary resuscitation must be continued throughout and after the operation as this improves the prognosis for mother and child.[16] In the event of a successful outcome the patients should be transferred to their appropriate intensive care units as soon as clinical conditions permit so that their management after arrest can be continued.

> **Algorithm for resuscitation in late pregnancy**
>
> 1 Identify arrest
> 2 Start basic life support immediately with cricoid pressure, and inferior vena caval decompression (wedge or manual uterine displacement)
> 3 Assemble staff, equipment, and drugs for advanced life support
> 4 Advanced life support—defibrillation, adrenaline, etc
> 5 Proceed to surgical delivery if no response to 1–4 in five minutes, continuing advanced life support during and after delivery
> 6 Open chest cardiac massage if 1–5 are ineffective
> 7 Transfer to intensive treatment unit

Training

The key factor in successful resuscitation in late pregnancy is that all nursing and medical staff concerned with obstetric care are trained in cardiopulmonary resuscitation.

Retention of cardiopulmonary resuscitation skills has been shown to be poor,[17] particularly in staff such as midwives and obstetricians who fortunately have little opportunity to practise them.[4] Regular short periods of practice on a mannikin simulator are therefore essential, either with an instructor supervising or in a self retraining group. We recommend 10–15 minute periods of practice every six months.

Members of the public and the ambulance service should also be aware of the additional problems associated with resuscitation in late pregnancy. The training of ambulance staff in cardiopulmonary resuscitation in late pregnancy is of current interest as courses have been initiated in at least one health district (South Glamorgan) for extended training of ambulance staff. These trained staff (paramedics) will eventually be the primary responders to obstetric emergency calls in the community.

> **Midwives and obstetricians**
>
> Train in cardiopulmonary resuscitation
> Provide mannikins for practice
> Retrain periodically
>
> **Ambulance crews and members of the public**
>
> Inform about specific problems of resuscitating pregnant women suffering cardiac arrest

---

1 Turnbull AC, Tindall VR, Robson G, et al. Report on confidential enquiries into maternal deaths in England and Wales 1982–84. London: HMSO, 1989. (Department of Health and Social Security. Report on health and social subjects No 34).

2 Stokes IM. Myocardial infarction and cardiac arrest in the second trimester followed by assisted vaginal delivery under epidural analgesia at 38 weeks. Br J Obstet Gynaecol 1984;91:197–8.

3 Ueland K, Novy, MJ, Peterson EN, Metcalfe J. Maternal cardiovascular dynamics. IV. The influence of gestational age on the maternal cardiovascular response to posture and exercise. Am J Obstet Gynecol 1969;104:856–64.

4 Rees GAD, Willis BA. Resuscitation in late pregnancy. Anaesthesia 1988;43:347–9.

5 Chamberlain DA. Guidelines for cardiopulmonary resuscitation: advanced life support. Br Med J 1989; 299:446–8.

6 Caplan RA, Ward RJ, Posner K, Cheney FW. Unexpected cardiac arrest during spinal anesthesia: closed-claims analysis of predisposing factors. Anesthesiology 1988;68:5–11.

7 Kasten GW, Martin ST. Bupivicaine cardiovascular toxicity: comparison of treatment with bretylium and lidocaine. Anesth Analg 1985;64:911–16.

8 Marx GF. Cardiopulmonary resuscitation of late pregnant women. Anesthesiology 1982;56:156.

9 De Pace NL, Betesh SS, Kolter MN. "Post mortem" cesarean section with recovery of both mother and offspring. JAMA 1982;248:971–97.

10 Katz VL, Dotters D, Droegemueller W. Perimortem cesarean delivery. Obstet Gynecol 1986;68:571–6.

11 Lindsay SL, Hanson GC. Cardiac arrest in near-term pregnancy. Anaesthesia 1987; 42:1074–7.

12 Oates S, Williams GL, Rees GAD. Cardiopulmonary resuscitation in late pregnancy. Br Med J 1988;297:404–5.

13 Kerr MG, Scott DB, Samuel E. Studies of the inferior vena cava in late pregnancy. Br Med J 1964;i:532–3.

14 Archer GW, Marx GF. Arterial oxygen tension during apnoea in parturient women. Br J Anaesth 1974;46:358–60.

15 Weil AM, Graber VR. The management of the near-term pregnant patient who dies undelivered. Am J Obstet Gynecol 1957;73:754–8.

16 Weber, CE. Post mortem cesarean section: review of the literature case reports. Am J Obstet Gynecol 1971;110:158–65.

17 Marsden AK. Guidelines for cardiopulmonary resuscitation: basic life support. Br Med J 1989;299:442–5.

RESUSCITATION AT BIRTH

A D MILNER

The priority of all those responsible for the care of babies at birth must be to ensure that adequate resuscitation facilities are available. Sadly, some babies have irreversible brain damage by the time of delivery, but it is unacceptable that any damage should occur after delivery because equipment is inadequate or staff insufficiently trained.

All babies at increased risk should be delivered in a unit with full respiratory support facilities. These deliveries must always be attended by a doctor who is solely responsible for the care of the baby and skilled in resuscitation. Whenever possible there should also be a trained assistant who can provide additional help if necessary. The list of babies at increased risk is relatively long—they make up about 25% of all deliveries—and will include about two thirds of those requiring resuscitation. The remaining one third of resuscitations occur in babies born after a normal uneventful labour who have no apparent risk factors. Labour ward staff must therefore be able to provide adequate resuscitation until further help can be obtained.

High risk deliveries	
Delivery	*Fetal*
Fetal distress	Multiple pregnancy
Abnormal presentation	Preterm
Prolapsed cord	Small for dates
Antepartum	Rhesus isoimmunisation
haemorrhage	Abnormal baby
Meconium staining	
High forceps	
Maternal	*Obstetrician*
Heavy sedation	Worried!
Drug addiction	
Diabetes	
Chronic illness	

Equipment

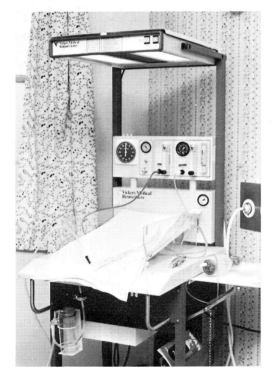

The padded platform on which the baby is nursed can be either flat or have a head down tilt. Wall mounting is satisfactory and certainly cheaper than the trolley models, provided, of course, that a unit is available for each delivery area. It is essential to have an overhead heater with an output of 3–500 watts, mounted about 1 metre above the platform. This must have a manual control as servo systems are slow to set up and likely to malfunction when the baby's skin is wet. These heaters are essential, as even in environments of 20–24°C the core temperature of an asphyxiated wet baby can drop by 5°C in as many minutes. Facilities must be available for manual face mask resuscitation, endotracheal tube resuscitation, and umbilical vein catheterisation. Additional equipment includes an overhead light, a clock with a second hand, suction equipment, a stethoscope, and preferably an electrocardiographic monitor.

Equipment for resuscitation		
Padded shelf	Clock	Face mask system
Overhead heater	Stethoscope	Endotracheal tube system
Overhead light	Electrocardiographic	(2·0–3·5 mm)
Oxygen cylinder (±wall	monitor	Umbilical vein catheter set
supply)	Laryngoscope	Syringes—1, 10, 20 ml
Suctions		
(50–100 cm H₂O)		

Procedure at delivery

In most units it is standard policy to suck out the pharynx as soon as the face appears, using a suction catheter. This is almost always unnecessary, unless the amniotic fluid is stained with meconium or blood. Aggressive pharyngeal suction can also delay the onset of spontaneous respiration for a considerable time. Once the baby is delivered the attendant should wipe any excess fluid off the baby, using a warm towel to reduce evaporative heat loss, at the same time examining the child for major external congenital abnormalities, such as spina bifida and severe microcephaly. Most babies will start breathing during this period, as the median time for the onset of spontaneous respiration is only 10 seconds. They can then be handed to their parents. If necessary the baby can be encouraged to breathe by skin stimulation—for example, flicking the baby's feet. Those not responding must be transferred immediately to the Resuscitaire.

Resuscitation procedure

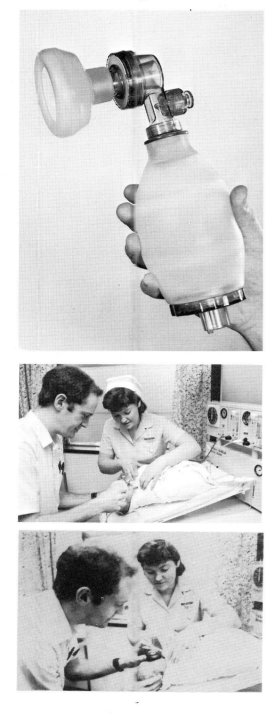

Check first for respiratory efforts. If these are present and perhaps vigorous but producing no tidal exchange the airway is obstructed. This can often be overcome by extending the baby's neck. If the baby has choanal atresia or Pierre Robin syndrome (cleft palate and micrognathia) obstruction will continue until an airway is inserted.

If respiratory efforts are feeble or totally absent count the heart rate for 10–15 seconds using the stethoscope. When the heart rate is over 80 beats/minute it is sufficient to repeat skin stimulation and if this fails to proceed to face mask resuscitation.

Face mask resuscitation—Only face masks consisting of a soft continuous ring provide an adequate seal. Most standard neonatal manual resuscitation devices fail to produce adequate tidal exchange when the pressure limiting device is unimpeded. Thus a satisfactory outcome almost always depends on the inflation pressure stimulating the baby to make inspiratory efforts (Head's paradoxical reflex). This poor performance is related to the short inspiratory time (one third to half a second) provided by the devices. Tidal exchange can be increased by using a 500 ml rather than a standard 250 ml reservoir, which allows inflation pressure to be maintained for one second.

More satisfactory tidal exchange can be achieved by bleeding oxygen directly into the face mask at 4–6 l/minute and occluding the outlet from the face mask as if it were an endotracheal T piece. Obviously it is essential to incorporate a pressure valve into the inspiratory lines so that the pressures cannot exceed 30 cm H_2O. The baby's lungs can then be inflated at rates of about 30/minute, allowing 1 second for each part of the cycle. Listen to the baby's chest within 5–10 inflations to check that there is bilateral air entry and that the heart rate is satisfactory. If the heart rate falls below 80 beats/minute proceed immediately to endotracheal intubation.

Endotracheal intubation—Most non-anaesthetists find a straight bladed laryngoscope preferable for performing intubation. This must be held in the left hand and the baby's neck gently extended, if necessary by the assistant. Pass the laryngoscope down, making sure that it is in the mid line, until the epiglottis comes into view. The tip of the blade can then be positioned either proximal to or immediately over the epiglottis so that the cords are brought into view. Gentle backward pressure may need to be applied over the larynx at this stage. As the airway tends to be filled with fluid, the upper airway may have to be cleared with the suction catheter held in the right hand.

Once the cords are visible pass the endotracheal tube, using the right hand, and remove the laryngoscope blade, taking care that this does not displace the tube out of the larynx. Then attach the endotracheal tube either to a T piece system, incorporating a 30–40 cm H_2O blow off valve in the inspiratory line, or to a neonatal manual resuscitation device. If a T piece is used maintain the initial inflation pressure for two to three seconds, which will help lung expansion. The baby can subsequently be ventilated at a rate of 30/minute, allowing about 1 second for each inflation.

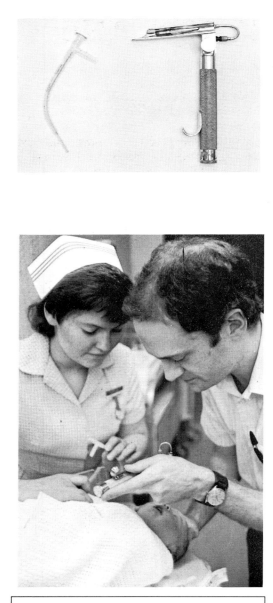

Inspect the chest during the first few inflations, looking for evidence of chest wall movement, and confirm by auscultation that oxygen is entering both lungs. If there is no air entry the most likely cause is that the endotracheal tube is lying in the oesophagus. If this is suspected remove the endotracheal tube immediately and reintubate. If auscultation shows that oxygen is entering one lung only, usually the right, try withdrawing the endotracheal tube by 1 cm while listening over the left lung. If this leads to dramatic improvement the tip of the endotracheal tube was lying in the right main bronchus. If there is no improvement the possible causes include pneumothorax, diaphragmatic hernia, or pleural effusion.

Severe bradycardia—If the heart rate falls below 30 beats/minute external cardiac massage must be started by compression over the junction of the lower and middle third of the sternum, using the tips of two fingers or by placing a hand round the chest and compressing it between the thumb and fingers at a rate of 100–120 compressions a minute. This will achieve about three compressions for every ventilation. If there is no dramatic improvement within 10–15 seconds the umbilical vein should be catheterised using a 5 French gauge catheter. This is best achieved by transecting the cord 2–3 cm away from the abdominal skin and inserting a catheter until there is a free flow of blood up the catheter. The baby should then be given 3 mmol of sodium bicarbonate per kg body weight over two to three minutes. This is best provided by mixing 8·4% solution mixed with an equal volume of 10% destrose, injecting a total of 20 ml to a term baby and 10 ml to a small baby, while continuing external cardiac massage and intermittent positive pressure ventilation. Those who fail to respond or who are in asystole require 1 ml adrenaline 1 in 10 000. This can be given either intravenously or injected directly down the endotracheal tube.

It is reasonable to continue with this regimen for 20 minutes, even in those who are born in apparent asystole, provided that a fetal heart beat was noted within 15 minutes of delivery. Resuscitation efforts should not be continued beyond half an hour unless the baby is making at least intermittent respiratory efforts.

Intravenous naloxone (40 µg) should be given to all babies who become pink and have an obviously satisfactory circulation on resuscitation but fail to start adequate respiratory efforts. There is often a history of recent maternal opiate sedation. Some authorities recommend that an additional 200 µg should be given intramuscularly to prevent relapse.

Meconium aspiration—Direct laryngoscopy should be carried out immediately after birth whenever there is meconium staining. If this shows meconium in the pharynx and trachea intubate the child immediately and attach the side port of the endotracheal tube to the suction source. Then suck up the free fluid while removing the endotracheal tube and then reintubate. Provided the baby's heart rate remains about 60 beats/minute this procedure can be repeated until meconium is no longer recovered. The use of direct mouth suction or even oral mucous extractors has been discouraged since infection with human immuodeficiency virus (HIV) was established as occurring congenitally.

Drugs for emergency use	
Sodium bicarbonate	8·4%
Dextrose	10%
Adrenaline	1 in 10 000
Naloxone	200 µg

Preterm resuscitation

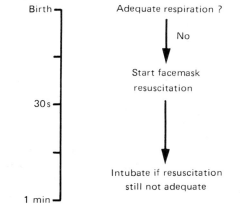

Babies with a gestation of more than 32 weeks do not differ from full term babies in their requirement for resuscitation. At less than this gestation they may have a lower morbidity and mortality if a more active intervention policy is adopted. There is, however, no evidence that a rigid policy whereby all babies with a gestation of less than 28 or 30 weeks are routinely intubated leads to improved outcome. Indeed, unless the operator is extremely skilful, intervention may produce severe hypoxia in a previously lively pink baby and produce conditions that may well predispose to intraventricular haemorrhage. A reasonable compromise would therefore seem to be to start face mask resuscitation at 15–30 seconds unless the baby has entirely adequate respiratory efforts and to proceed to intubation if the baby has not achieved satisfactory respiratory efforts by 30–60 seconds.

RESUSCITATION OF INFANTS AND CHILDREN

D A ZIDEMAN

In 1987 in England and Wales 6272 infants died aged under one year (9·2 per 1000 live births); 2684 of these deaths occurred in the first week of life and 3448 in the first month. (Although these statistics include infants dying at birth, delivery room resuscitation has a different aetiology and in most cases should be a planned event. It is considered separately in another chapter).

During the same period 11·3% of deaths in children aged 28 days to 14 years were due to accidental causes (32% of deaths in the 5–14 age group). If most of these children are considered to have been fit and healthy before their accident it is surprising that paediatric resuscitation does not play a more prominent part in community and hospital resuscitation programmes.

Hypoxia is the most common cause of cardiac arrest in infants and children. Sudden infant death syndrome; the loss of blood or body fluids, as in gastroenteritis and resulting in circulatory hypovolaemia; congenital heart disease; and septicaemia are also notable causes. Treatment must be immediate to be effective; delays in recognising or treating a cardiac arrest or therapeutic mistakes may seriously affect the outcome.

Hypoxia
Sudden infant death syndrome
Loss of blood and bodily fluids
Congenital heart disease
Septicaemia

Basic life support

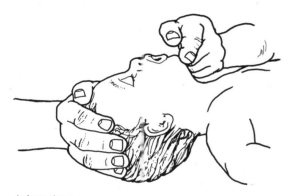

Infant airway

Resuscitation must begin immediately and should not await the arrival of equipment. This is essential in infants and children as just the simple manoeuvre of opening the airway may be all that is needed and may certainly prevent any further progress of the event.

As in any resuscitation, the airway, breathing, circulation sequence is most appropriate.

Airway

Opening the airway is achieved by tilting the head and supporting the lower jaw.

Care must be taken: (a) not to overextend the neck as this may cause the soft trachea to kink and obstruct, and (b) not to press on the soft tissues in the floor of the mouth. Pressure in this area will force the tongue into the airway and cause obstruction.

The small infant is an obligatory nose breather so the patency of the nasal passages must be checked and maintained.

Maintaining the paediatric airway is a matter of trying various positions until the most satisfactory one is found. The rescuer must be flexible and willing to adapt his technique. The obstructed airway in infants and children is one example of a cause of collapse which is often immediately treatable. Obstruction may be caused by a foreign body (food or a toy) or by vomit. Careful removal of a foreign body is essential so as not to make the situation worse. An indifferent technique, such as blind probing or finger sweeps, may result in trauma, haemorrhage, and oedema of the upper airway or further impaction of the foreign body. Inverting the child and applying back blows is an effective way of clearing an obstruction. The abdominal thrust procedure can be applied to children aged over 5.

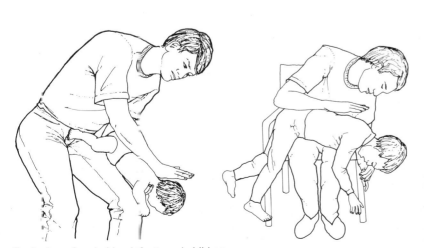

Back blows for choking infants and children

57

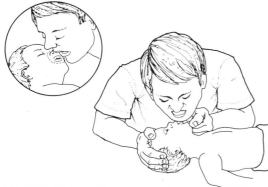

Mouth to mouth and nose ventilation

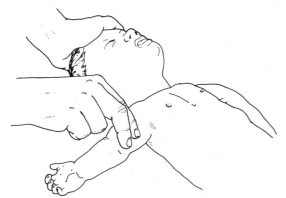

Brachial pulse in infants

	Baby	Child
Heart rate (beats/min)	120	100
External chest compressions/min	120	100
Depth (cm)	1–1½	2–3
Respiratory rate (breaths/min)	37	20
Expired air resuscitation/min	24	20

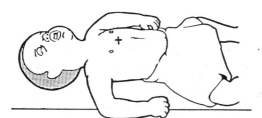

Chest compression position

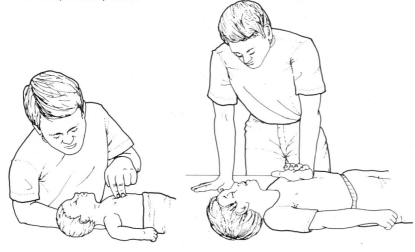

Chest compression in infants and children

Infectious diseases of the upper airway may cause serious and even fatal obstruction if not dealt with properly. The term croup is used to describe such diseases and is simply diagnosed as an inspiratory stridor. The child may prefer to sit up and lean forward. Breathing a humidified atmosphere may also help, but further active interference may lead to a rapid worsening of the condition. These children must be moved, with care and supervision, into hospital to be dealt with by an expert team with the proper equipment.

Breathing

The patency of the airway is checked by listening and feeling for breaths over the nose and mouth of the child. The rescuer must look to see if the child has normal chest movements or if there is intercostal recession or a see-saw movement of the chest or abdomen, indicating residual airway obstruction. Small children may also show flaring of the nares.

Expired air resuscitation must be started immediately if the child is not breathing. With the airway held open, the rescuer should cover the child's mouth (or mouth and nose) with his mouth and breathe gently into the child until the chest rises. The correct volume can be simply judged by watching the chest movement. Ventilation may be increased by raising the rate of breathing and not by increasing the tidal volume.

Four individual breaths should be given initially. If the child requires only ventilation then breathing is continued at a rate of 15 to 30 breaths a minute according to the size of the child.

Circulation

The circulation is best assessed by palpating the brachial pulse [1] The femoral or carotid pulses may also be used depending on the experience of the rescuer. The pulse should be assessed not only for adequacy of volume but also for heart rate. Bradycardias occasionally accompany hypoxia, and they are best treated by establishing adequate ventilation. Knowledge of the relevant pulse rates of infants and children is essential to make this diagnosis.

If an adequate pulse is not found external chest compressions must be started. The heart lies under the lower part of the sternum in children and thus chest compressions should be applied to the junction of the lower and middle third of the sternum.[2] The optimal position is found by measuring either one finger breadth below the internipple line or the same distance above the xiphisternum.[3] The method of applying chest compressions depends on the child's size.

The small baby is best served by encircling the baby's chest with both hands; the sternum is compressed by the thumbs and additional support provided by the interlaced fingers behind the infant's back. In toddlers and small children compressions can be applied by the tips of two fingers, while the larger child may require compressions applied by the heel of one hand.

The rate and depth of compressions also depends on the child's size. Compressions should be smooth and the compression phase last at least half the cycle. The accuracy of the rate and depth of compression is not vitally important; again the rescuer should be flexible and able to adapt his technique to achieve the best result. The rate of compressions should be fast enough to provide a circulation, the depth of compression deep enough to feel a pulse on palpation. Although the ideal is to match the normal physiological rates, a compression rate of at least 100 per minute is recommended.

A ratio of five compressions to one ventilation is recommended for infants and children. It is essential that adequate ventilation be achieved and a pause in the chest compressions may be required to ensure this. The adult ratio of two ventilations to 15 compressions should be used in older children.

Advanced life support

Age	Endotracheal tube interna diameter (mm)	Length (cm)		Suction catheter (F)
		Oral	Nasal	
Premature	2·5–3·C	11	13·5	6
Newborn	3·5	12	14	8
1 Year	4·0	13	15	8
2 Years	4·5	14	16	8
4 Years	5·0	15	17	10
6 Years	5·5	17	19	10
8 Years	6·0	19	21	10
10 Years	6·5	20	22	10
12 Years	7·0	21	22	10
14 Years	7·5	22	23	10
16 Years	8·0	23	24	12

Age and weight	Bag volume (ml)	Tidal volume (ml)
<2 years (<7 kg)	240	205
2–10 years (7–30 kg)	500	350
>10 years (>30 kg)	1600	1000

Paediatric masks

The use of equipment in paediatric resuscitation is fraught with difficulties. Not only must a wide range of equipment be available to correspond with the variety of sizes of child but also the rescuer must be skilled enough to be able to choose and use the equipment efficiently.

Airway

The simplest airway adjunct is the Guedel oropharyngeal airway, but even here there is a choice of sizes from 000 to 4. Too small an airway will not overcome the obstruction of the tongue and may force it to the back of the pharynx. Too large an airway may injure the posterior pharyngeal wall. Nasopharyngeal airways are often a simple solution in children—for example, an endotracheal tube of suitable nasal diameter cut to a short length.

If the paediatric airway is to be guaranteed the child must be intubated. Intubation requires skill acquired only through training and practice. A complete range of sizes of endotracheal tubes must be available, and the choice is made by using either a table or a simple formula. The endotracheal tube must be cut to an appropriate length and after intubation the position of the tip of the tube should be checked by auscultation to ensure that the left or right main bronchi have not been inadvertently entered, resulting in the ventilation of one lung only.

Once the tube is correctly positioned it should be firmly secured to prevent accidental movement or inadvertent extubation.

There is a wide variety of ancillary intubation equipment. The straight blade laryngoscope is usually recommended for infants and children but in emergencies an adult curved blade can be used with extreme care. There is also a choice of endotracheal tube connections. The simplest answer is to pick the system which fits most of the ventilation equipment available. In the majority of cases this will be the 15 mm British standard connector. A range of sizes of suction catheters must also be available to keep the airway clear.

Breathing

Supplemental oxygen by facemask, head box, nasal cannulae, or an oxygen tent is a simple and useful initial solution. If the child is not breathing then ventilation can be achieved with a resuscitation bag attached to a mask or an endotracheal tube.

The resuscitation bags usually used are self inflating and made in three sizes. The two smaller bags have a pressure limiting device preset to 45cm H_2O to prevent overpressurisation of the child's lungs. This can be overridden where the lungs have become non-compliant. Spontaneous respiration is possible through such bags. It is always worth adding supplemental oxygen to a resuscitation bag. In more experienced hands the Jackson Rees modification of the Ayres T piece is more adaptable, but, not being self inflating, this requires a reliable and controllable gas supply.

There are a variety of designs and sizes of masks to be used in association with a resuscitation bag. The Rendell-Baker design is often favoured as its shape minimises apparatus dead space, but more recently circular masks, made of soft plastic, have been found to be successful, especially by inexperienced users. A snug fit is essential when selecting the size of mask. Clear plastic masks are recommended so that the child's colour can be observed without having to remove the mask during resuscitation.

Automatic resuscitators are, at present, not recommended for use with children. Paediatric ventilation requires repeated re-evaluation and adaptation of techniques, and a false sense of security may be developed which can result in inadequate or excessive ventilation.

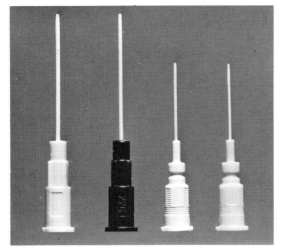

Intravenous cannulae (20–26 standard wire gauge)

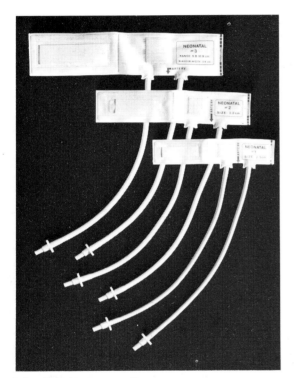

Infant blood pressure cuffs

Circulation

The administration of fluids and drugs to support the circulation usually requires intravenous access. Fluids can be administered via the interosseous route and some drugs can be given down the endotracheal tube for absorption in the lungs. If the latter route is used a short period of hyperventilation is required to aid distribution and absorption of the drug by the pulmonary vascular bed.

One of the major problems in paediatric resuscitation is establishing intravenous access. The choice of which cannula to use and what route to select is a matter of personal preference and experience. Central venous access is better than peripheral access because of the poor peripheral blood flow during resuscitation. Central venous access may be gained via the femoral, subclavian, or internal or external jugular veins. Whichever route is chosen, central or peripheral, it must be remembered that it is the venous access which is important and not the size of the cannula. Most resuscitations can be carried out by drug administration through a 20 or 22 standard wire gauge cannula.

Fluids should be administered sparingly as fluid overload can be a problem in resuscitation attempts. Peripheral venous administration often necessitates the flushing of drugs centrally Repeated administration via this route can easily result in fluid overload. A record of all fluids given either as drugs or as fluid loading should be maintained. In hypovolaemic conditions, such as trauma or gastroenteritis, it may be necessary to give blood, plasma, or a plasma substitute in appropriate volumes. Children do not tolerate hypovolaemia and the rescuer must bear in mind their normal circulating blood volume.

Heart rate and cardiac rhythm are best assessed by attaching the child to an electrocardiographic monitor. A stethoscope allows auscultation of the heart and breath sounds. Blood pressure measurements depend on using the right size of paediatric blood pressure cuff together with a machine capable of measuring young children's relatively low but normal blood pressures. The width of the cuff should be two thirds of the length of the child's upper arm.

Ventricular fibrillation and ventricular tachycardia are not often a problem in paediatric resuscitation. Should they occur defibrillation is the treatment of choice. Two joules/kg is the recommended energy level. Some defibrillators can be charged only to preset levels (20 50 100 200, or 400J) whereas others have a maximum output of 100 J when the paediatric paddles have been connected. The paddle size and position are chosen as being those which provide the best contact with the child's chest wall. Paddles are available in two sizes, 4·5 or 8 cm in diameter.

Drugs

Drugs may be given intravenously or via the endotracheal tube. The correct dose requires knowledge of the recommended dose in mg/kg (surface areas are inappropriate in resuscitation). Thus the rescuer must know the body weight of the child. Most children who have been admitted to hospital before the resuscitation attempt have usually been weighed. If the child is particularly ill and likely to need cardiopulmonary resuscitation the drug doses should be precalculated both in mg of drug required and in ml of drug solution to be administered.

Drug	Dose	Route
Adrenaline	10 µg/kg (0·1 ml/kg of 1 in 10 000)	Intravenous or endotracheal
Atropine	0·02 mg/kg (maximum 0·6 mg)	Intravenous or endotracheal
Sodium bicarbonate	1 mmol/kg (1 ml/kg of 8·4%)	Intravenous
Calcium chloride	5–10 mg/kg (0·3 ml/kg of 10%)	Intravenous
Lignocaine	1 mg/kg (0·1 ml/kg of 1%)	Intravenous or endotracheal
Dextrose	1 g/kg (2 ml/kg of 50%)	
Frusemide	1 mg/kg	

Infusions (usually in 5% dextrose solution)

Adrenaline—0·02 to 0·05 µg/kg/min

Isoprenaline—0·05 to 0·1 µg/kg/min

Dopamine—1–10 µg/kg/min (calculate by adding 3×bodyweight in mg of dopamine to 50 ml of 5% dextrose—infusion in ml/h equivalent to µg/kg/min)

Simple mistakes in calculating dosages or the conversion of drug doses to millilitres of solution to be administered can have fatal consequences.

> Infants double their birthweight in 5 months
>
> Infants treble their birthweight in 1 year
>
> Aged 1–9 years weight (kg) = (age + 4) × 2
>
> Aged 7–12 years weight (kg) = age × 3

> Ventilation
>
> Electrocardiograph
>
> Arterial and venous pressure monitoring
>
> Chest radiograph
>
> Plasma electrolytes and glucose
>
> Arterial pH and blood gases

1 Cavallaro DL, Melko RJ. Comparison of two techniques for detecting cardiac activity in infants. *Crit Care Med* 1983;11:189–90.
2 Phillips GWL, Zideman DA. Relation of infant heart to sternum: Its significance in cardiopulmonary resuscitation. *Lancet* 1986;i:1024–5.
3 Orlowski JP. Optimum position for external cardiac compression in infants and young children. *Ann Emerg Med* 1986;15:667–73.

Further reading

Ludwig S, Kettrick RG. Pediatric resuscitation for the non-pediatrician. In: Jacobson S, ed. *Clinics in emergency medicine. Resuscitation.* Vol 2. Edinburgh: Churchill Livingstone, 1983:101–2.
Bray RJ. The management of cardiac arrest in infants and children. *Br J Hosp Med* 1985;34:72–81.
Zideman DA. Resuscitation in paediatrics. In: Sumner F, Hatch DJ, eds. *Clinics in anaesthesiology. Paediatric anaesthesia.* Vol 3, No 3. London: WB Saunders, 1985: 765–83.

In an emergency the child may not present with a known accurate body weight. It is usually easier to obtain or estimate the child's age, and the weight can then be estimated by using a paediatric nomogram. An alternative is to use the accompanying approximate rules of thumb.

The simplest solution is to use a table that relates age, weight, and drug dosage or to use a paediatric resuscitation chart relating age, weight, and length (see below).

Temperature

It is vitally important to maintain or restore the child's body temperature during resuscitation. Hypothermia causes additional strain on the cardiovascular system. Warm blankets, infrared heaters, and incubators should all be available as part of the paediatric resuscitation equipment.

Care after resuscitation

Like adults, children require intensive postresuscitation care. Ventilation may be needed, and monitoring of the arterial and central venous pressures may require invasive techniques. Investigations should include a chest radiograph and measurement of plasma electrolyte and blood sugar concentrations. Arterial pH and blood gases may indicate a cause of the collapse and require further correction to prevent a recurrence.

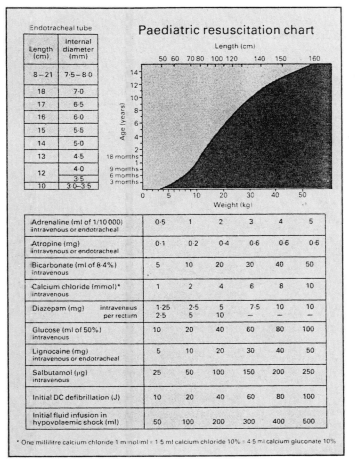

The graph represents age plotted against weight for the 50th centile boy-girl average. To the left are shown dimensions of endotracheal tubes, which correlate well with age. Below is a table showing various drug doses for use in cardiorespiratory arrest or other urgent conditions. Also included are defibrillator settings and suggestions for initial fluid infusion in hypovolaemia. The doses comply with the present Resuscitation Council guidelines. If the weight is already known drug dosage may be estimated by moving directly downwards from the weight axis. If age but not weight is known dosage may be estimated by tracing across the graph and then down to the dose. If neither is known a rapid stretched out length may be measured with a tape measure and the non-linear scale above the graph used to estimate drug dosage.

From: Oakley PA. Inaccuracy and delay in decision making in paediatric resuscitation, and a proposed reference chart to reduce error. *Br Med J* 1988;**297**:817–19.
Based on the guidelines of the Resuscitation Council (UK).

Copies of the chart are available from the British Medical Journal either as posters or as postcards. Please write for details.

DROWNING AND NEAR DROWNING

MARK HARRIES

Definition and incidence

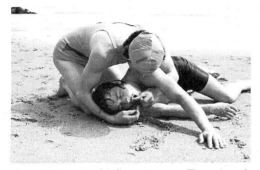

Clearing the airway with finger sweeps. The value of abdominal thrusts or back blows remains to be proved.

Drowning is defined as death by asphyxia caused by submersion in a fluid and near drowning as survival from asphyxia caused in this way. The yearly incidence of drowning ranges from 0·4 to 0·9 deaths per 100 000 and is highest in temperate and in under developed countries. The incidence of near drowning is not known. In Britain around 700 people drown each year, a figure that has changed little in 30 years. Overall men who die by drowning outnumber women by over 4 to 1, but in the age range 15 to 25 men are 10 times more likely to die. Two thirds of all fatalities occur in fresh water because rescue services tend to be more sparse on inland waters than they are on the coast and not, as is sometimes believed, because fresh water is any more lethal than salt. About 20% of adults who die show evidence of recent alcohol ingestion.

Clinical features and management

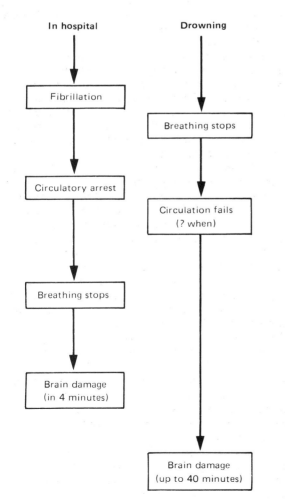

Patients present with acute hypothermia and hypoxia. Cerebral injury results if the hypoxia is not treated promptly, and in addition aspirated water causes lung injury. Management is complex and best divided into care that can be provided under difficult circumstances in the field and care that can be given later.

Management in the field

About 70% of patients who reach hospital apnoeic but with a detectable pulse can be expected to survive. By contrast only 8% survive if the heart cannot be restarted in the field. Effective cardiopulmonary resuscitation is essential and should be uninterrupted from the time of rescue to arrival in hospital. Cardiopulmonary arrest, such as is seen after myocardial infarction, does not occur in drowning. What occurs is respiratory and then cardiac arrest; the events are reversed, and perfusion of the brain continues probably for some time after submersion. This might explain why some people have been revived without apparent brain damage after total submersion for more than 40 minutes.

The airway—The mouth is best cleared with a single finger sweep that leaves well fitting dentures in place but removes loose foreign bodies. Unless difficulty is encountered with inflating the chest, drainage manoeuvres are probably a waste of time. Over half the victims of immersion vomit during resuscitation, and the rescuer must be ready to turn the patient promptly to prevent aspiration of vomit.

Breathing—Most survivors are found to be hypoxic on arrival in hospital. Oxygen must be given as early as possible after rescue. Patients who are already breathing should be allowed to breathe oxygen delivered through a loosely fitting mask at a flow rate of 8 l/minute. Oxygen concentrations of up to 40% can be given in this way. Such patients should be kept in the lateral or recovery position during treatment.

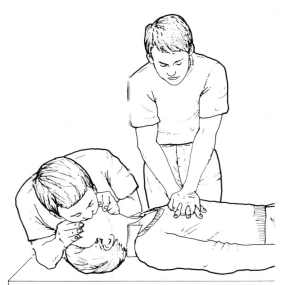

Heart and lung resuscitation (two rescuers)

Carotid pulse

Patients who are not breathing should ideally be intubated and ventilated. In this way almost 100% oxygen can be given and the airway is secured in the event of vomiting. The ideal is seldom possible in the field, so mouth to mouth resuscitation is given first, then, as the equipment becomes available, mouth to mask and then to bag mask with a Guedel airway. The highest concentrations of oxygen can only be reached with the addition of a reservoir bag. The colour of the lips of patients who are cold provides no guidance to the level of oxygenation.

Circulation—Palpation of the carotid pulse is difficult in the field, especially if the patient happens to be cold, in which case the pulse can be feeble, very slow, and irregular. Only if the pulse is absent should chest compression be applied because of the risk of precipitating ventricular fibrillation.

Profoundly hypothermic pulseless patients have been revived after more than two hours of chest compression.

It is usually better to try to stabilise the patient's condition at the accident site rather than to attempt to do so under more difficult circumstances in transit.

Management in hospital

Fully conscious patient—Any patient who may have inhaled water should undergo arterial gas measurement and chest radiography. If rewarming is necessary it is best done in bath water at 40°C. Discharge from hospital is safe after a patient has been observed for six hours provided that:
(a) The arterial oxygen is normal when the patient is breathing air
(b) The chest x ray is clear
(c) No lung crackles are audible on auscultation
(d) No cough persists
(e) There is no fever

Patient unwell but breathing—In addition to the observations already mentioned, these patients require cardiac monitoring and the measurement of core temperature using a low reading rectal probe. Rewarming is achieved by passive means, by insulating in thick blankets, after removing wet clothing. Hypoxia should be treated with oxygen delivered at 8 l/minute. The risk of vomiting is high, so the patient should be nursed in the lateral position.

Apnoeic patient with a pulse—An endotracheal tube should be inserted if this has not already been done. Oxygen can then be given at the highest possible concentration and the lungs are protected against the risk of aspiration. Blood should be drawn for culture, white cell count, and estimation of serum electrolytes. Plasma expansion is often required and although the choice of fluid is not critical, sodium bicarbonate should be avoided if possible. A central venous route has the added advantage of allowing simultaneous assessment of venous pressure.

Apnoeic pulseless patient—Circulation is supported by chest compression that may have to continue for an hour or more. Ventricular fibrillation develops as a consequence of hypothermia and responds poorly to cardioversion until the core temperature rises. This can be accelerated with active rewarming by heating the blood on bypass. Nodal bradyarrhythmias are probably best left untreated as the patient warms up.

Clinical state of patient	Investigations	Management
Fully conscious	Blood gases Chest x ray	Allow home after six hours if: (a) Normal gases (b) Normal chest x ray (c) No lung crackles (d) No cough (e) No fever
Unwell but breathing	Blood gases Chest x ray Cardiac monitor Rectal temperature	Oxygen at 8 l/minute. Rewarm in woollen blankets after removing wet clothes Nurse in the lateral position
Apnoeic with a pulse	Blood gases Chest x ray Cardiac monitor Rectal temperature Blood: Culture Cell count Electrolytes	Insert endotracheal tube Ventilate, if necessary with positive end expiratory pressure ventilation Insert intravenous line Plasma expansion
Apnoeic and pulseless	All the above	Continue chest compression during rewarming Consider rewarming on bypass

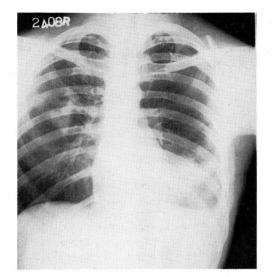

Shadowing in the left lower zone and right mid zone represents aspirated water. The patient is at risk of developing adult respiratory distress syndrome.

Late complications

Pulmonary oedema—The adult respiratory distress syndrome results from aspirating either fresh or salt water and has been recorded even in people who appear to be quite well after being rescued. The symptoms may be very rapid in onset, appearing within minutes of recovery from the water, but seldom start after more than four hours without some warning signs; these are:–

(a) A falling PaO_2 despite breathing oxygen,

(b) Shadows on the chest *x* ray,

(c) Lung crackles on auscultation.

The adult respiratory distress syndrome is treated with positive end expiratory pressure ventilation. Systemic steroids have not been shown to reduce lung injury and, because they may either mask or impair the response to infection, their use is not recommended.

Cerebral oedema—Cerebral oedema develops as a result of hypoxia as the patient warms up. Measurements of intracranial pressure have been made in children, in whom values of more than 20 mmHg give a poor prognosis. Attempts to reduce pressure with barbiturates and mechanical hyperventilation have not improved outcome. While the patient is still hypothermic the extent of brain damage cannot be estimated with any certainty.

Septicaemia—Fever is common in the first few hours, but systemic infection is a probable cause if fever occurs after 24 hours, particularly in the presence of neutropenia. Blood cultures should be taken before starting to give intravenous antibiotics, which should be effective against Gram negative organisms.

AIDS, HEPATITIS, AND RESUSCITATION

D A ZIDEMAN

In cardiopulmonary resuscitation there is no reason to delay basic life support (airway, breathing, and circulation) until the possible infective state of the patient has been established. A great deal has been written, by knowledgeable authors and by others, about the risks of contact of health care workers, resuscitators, first aiders, and the general public, with blood or body fluids of patients being resuscitated who are considered to be possible carriers of human immunodeficiency virus (HIV) or hepatitis B virus (HBV). In response to ill founded concern, prompted by the ill informed and the media, concerning the perceived risks of salivary exposure many "alternative methods" have been recommended.

Guidelines

A report from the Centers for Disease Control updated previous advice on universal precautions against parenteral, mucous membrane, or non-intact skin exposures to HIV or HBV.[1] It emphasised the fact that blood is the single most important source of these viruses and applied its recommendations for universal precaution to semen, vaginal secretions, and cerebrospinal, synovial, pleural, peritoneal, pericardial, and amniotic fluid and to any body fluid containing visible blood. Body fluids to which these universal precautions do not apply include sputum, nasal secretions, faeces, sweat, tears, urine, and vomit unless they contain visible blood. A series of epidemiological studies of the non-sexual contacts of patients with HIV suggested that the possibility of salivary transmission of HIV is remote,[2-6] and a further study showed that hepatitis B was not transmitted from resuscitation manikins.[7]

Protective airway devices

Despite the above, some health care workers and members of the general public may feel the need for some interpositional airway device, for example in accident departments when the saliva of trauma victims may be contaminated with blood. Before selecting such a device the user must be satisfied that it will function effectively in its resuscitation and protective roles and must be properly trained in its use, regularly tested in its use, properly informed about its cleaning, sterilisation, and disposal, and must be assured of its immediate availability at times of cardiopulmonary resuscitation.

Needlestick injuries

Resuscitation is an emergency procedure that does include, in its advanced stages, invasive techniques. Special care must be taken to ensure that, in the hustle and bustle of resuscitation, members of the resuscitation team are not accidentally contaminated with possibly infected material and are carefully guarded against needlestick and "sharp" injuries. Sharp disposal boxes should be part of resuscitation equipment. The decision about how many more of the recommended universal precautions should be applied should be based on the prevalence of HIV and HBV in the locality.

Training manikins

Practice in resuscitation techniques is an essential part of establishing an effective resuscitation service. Resuscitation training manikins have not been shown to be sources of virus infection. Nevertheless, sensible precautions must be taken to minimise potential cross infection, and the manikins must be formally disinfected after each use according to the manufacturers' recommendations.

Conclusion

Interpositional airway adjuncts are not essential for performing mouth to mouth resuscitation but, if a patient's oral cavity or saliva is contaminated with visible blood, using an adjunct can reassure the rescuer. Starting mouth to mouth respiration must not be delayed until such an airway adjunct is provided.

1 Centers for Disease Control. Update: universal precautions for prevention of transmission of human immunodeficiency virus, hepatitis B virus and other blood-borne pathogens in health care settings. *MMWR* 1988; **37:** 377–88.
2 Centers for Disease Control. Update: acquired immunodeficiency syndrome and human immunodeficiency virus infection among health care workers. *MMWR* 1988; **37:** 229–34, 239.
3 Friedland GH, Saltzman BR, Rogers MF, *et al.* Lack of transmission of HTLV-III/LAV infection to household contacts of patients with AIDS or AIDS related complex with oral candidiasis. *N Engl J Med* 1986; **314:** 344–9.
4 Jason JM, McDougal JS, Dixon G, *et al.* HTLV III-LAV antibody and immune status of household contacts and sexual partners of persons with hemophilia. *JAMA* 1986; **255:** 212–5.
5 Curran JW, Jaffe HW, Hardy AM, *et al.* Epidemiology of HIV infection and AIDS in the United States. *Science* 1988; **239:** 610–6.
6 Lifson AR. Do alternative modes for transmission of human immunodeficiency virus exist? A review. *JAMA* 1988; **259:** 1353–6.
7 Glaser JB, Nadler JP. Hepatitis B virus in a cardiopulmonary resuscitation training course: risk of transmission from a surface antigen-positive participant. *Arch Intern Med* 1985; **145:** 1653–5.

THE ETHICS OF RESUSCITATION

PETER J F BASKETT

Present day knowledge, skill, pharmacy, and technology have proved effective in prolonging useful life for many patients. Countless thousands have good reason to be thankful for cardiopulmonary resuscitation, and the numbers rise daily. Yet, in the wake of this advance, there is a small but important shadow of bizarre and distressing problems. These problems must be freely and openly addressed if we are to avoid criticism from others and from our own consciences.

Resuscitation attempts in the mortally ill do not enhance the dignity and serenity that we hope for our relatives and ourselves when we die. All too often resuscitation is begun in patients already destined for life as cardiac or respiratory cripples or who are suffering the terminal misery of untreatable cancer. From time to time, but fortunately rarely, resuscitation efforts may help to create the ultimate tragedy—the human vegetable—as the heart is more tolerant than the brain to the insult of hypoxia.

Merely prolonging the process of dying

The reasons for these apparent errors of judgment are several. In a high proportion of cases, particularly those occurring outside hospital, the victim and his circumstances are unknown to the rescuer, who may well not be competent to assess whether resuscitation is appropriate or not in the particular individual. Sadly, through lack of communication, this state of affairs also occurs from time to time in hospital practice. A junior ward nurse, unless explicitly instructed not to do so, feels, not unreasonably, obliged to call the resuscitation team to any patient with cardiorespiratory arrest. She is not qualified to certify death. The team is often unaware of the patient's condition and prognosis and, because of the urgency of the situation, begins treatment first and asks questions afterwards.

Ideally, resuscitation should be attempted only in patients who have a very high chance of successful revival for a comfortable and contented existence. A study of published reports containing results of series of resuscitation attempts shows that this ideal is far from being attained. Typical figures include a 12% survival rate for one month in 1972,[1] a 14% survival to be discharged from hospital,[2] and, more recently, a discharge rate of 14% in 1982[3] and 21·3% in 1984.[4] De Bard, reviewing published reports in 1981, reported an overall discharge rate of 17%.[5] In each of these series a substantial number—usually about 50–60%—failed to respond to the initial resuscitation attempts. In many of these, particularly the younger patients, effort was clearly justified initially. The cause of the arrest was apparently myocardial ischaemia, and the outcome cannot be confidently predicted in any individual patient. However, some of the papers drew attention to the large proportion of patients in whom resuscitative efforts were inappropriate and unjustified. Sowden *et al* reported an incidence of 25% of cases in which resuscitation merely prolonged the process of dying.

> A 32 year old woman was admitted in a quadraplegic state due to a spinal injury incurred when she had thrown herself from the Clifton Suspension Bridge. She had made 18 previous attempts at suicide over the previous five years, sometimes by taking an overdose of tablets of various kinds and sometimes by cutting her wrists. She had been injecting herself with heroin for the past seven years and had no close relationships with her family and no close friends. During her stay of two days in the intensive care unit she developed pneumonia and died. A conscious decision not to provide artificial ventilation and resuscitation had been made beforehand.

Though assessments are undoubtedly easier in retrospect, there are clearly many cases in which the decision not to resuscitate might have been made before the event. As the number of deaths in hospital always exceeds the number of calls for resuscitation, a decision not to resuscitation is clearly being made in many instances. There is, however, much room for improvement.

Deciding not to resuscitate

The decision not to resuscitate revolves around many factors—the patient's own wishes, the opinion of a relative, who may be reporting the known wishes of a patient who cannot communicate, the patient's social environment, the patient's prognosis, and his ability to cope with disablement of one form or other. The decision should not revolve around doctors' pride.

The examples in the boxes may serve as food for thought on whether the value judgment was right or wrong.

Decisions on whether or not to resuscitate are generally made about each patient in the atmosphere of close clinical supervision prevalent in intensive care units of the UK, and the decision is then communicated to the resident medical and nursing staff. In the general wards, however, the potential situation in specific patients may not actually be discussed, and inappropriate resuscitation occurs by default. There is a reluctance to label a mentally alert patient, who is nevertheless terminally ill, "Not for resuscitation." There are, sadly, doctors who refuse to acknowledge that the patient has reached end stage disease, perhaps because they have spent so much time and effort in treating them. There are those who, having spent their career in hospital practice, cannot comprehend the difficulties for the severely disabled of an existence without adequate help in a poor and miserable social environment. There are those who fear medicolegal sanctions if they put their name to an instruction not to resuscitate.

In the UK the decision not to resuscitate in the general wards tends to be an individual and informal one made ultimately by the clinician looking after the patient, perhaps at the instigation of others, such as the nursing staff and his team colleagues. The clinician is not, however, obliged to consider or make such a decision, much as it might be beneficial in many cases.

Formal policies

At the Chedoke and McMaster Hospitals in Hamilton, Ontario, a formal policy about when not to resuscitate has been introduced on the advice of the medical advisory committee and at the instigation of the nursing staff, who were concerned at the varied practices occurring in the hospital.[6] The very comprehensive policy and guidelines require that before writing "Do not resuscitate" on the patient's notes, the clinician must consult the patient or his relatives and seek a second opinion from another colleague if the patient or his relatives wish it. Correctly, the order must be reviewed at regular intervals. The General Council of the Canadian Medical Association had previously indicated that it was ethical for a doctor to write such an order in the appropriate circumstances.[7]

Initially, the Canadian doctors were concerned about a number of points, particularly potential infringement by the hospital administration of their clinical freedom, as they saw it, fear of medicolegal recriminations, and worry that patients and their relatives might interpret the no resuscitation policy as the withdrawal of palliation and comforting measures and pain relief. However, after implementation of the policy most clinicians felt that on the whole it was beneficial to both patients and doctors.

"Do not resuscitate" policies in the United States also tend to be formal affairs with a strict protocol to be followed.[8] It is unlikely, however, that doctors in the UK would be willing, or indeed wise, to conform to rigid guidelines in such a delicate, sensitive, and personal issue. This attitude may reflect the fact that the British doctor, by and large, is more confident of his relationship with his patients than his transatlantic counterpart, and it may also reflect a different feeling of trust on the part of the British patient towards his doctor.

Nevertheless, some form of non-coercive flexible guidelines are undoubtedly helpful and serve as a reminder that the decision must be faced and made.

Below is an extract from the guidelines approved by the medical staff committee at Frenchay Hospital, Bristol, which has been in use for the past four years.

There can be no rules, every case must be considered individually and this decision should be reviewed as appropriate—this may be on a weekly, daily, or hourly basis.

The decision should be made *before* it is needed and in many patients this will be *on* admission.

A decision to "DO NOT RESUSCITATE", IS ABSOLUTELY COMPATIBLE WITH CONTINUING MAXIMUM THERAPEUTIC AND NURSING CARE.
(1) Where the patient is competent (ie mentally fit and conscious), the decision "DO NOT RESUSCITATE" should be discussed where possible with the patient. This will not always be appropriate but, particularly in those patients with a slow progressive deterioration, it is important to *consider* it.
(2) If the patient is not competent to make such decisions, the appropriate family members should be consulted.
(3) Factors which may influence the decision to be made should include:—
   (a) Quality of life prior to this illness (highly subjective and only truly known to the patient himself).
   (b) Expected quality of life (medical and social) assuming recovery from this particular illness.
   (c) Likelihood of resuscitation being successful.
If at any time patients or their relatives request an attempt at resuscitation contrary to medical opinion—this should be carried out.

The decision to "DO NOT RESUSCITATE" should be recorded clearly in medical and nursing notes, signed, dated, and should be reviewed at appropriate intervals.

During the period of clinical use there have been no objections to the guidelines from either the medical or nursing staff.

A 62 year old woman had a cardiac arrest in a thoracic ward two days after undergoing pneumonectomy for resectable lung cancer. Her remaining lung was clearly fibrotic and malfunctioning and her cardiac arrest was probably hypoxic and hypercarbic in origin. Because no instructions had been given to the contrary, she was resuscitated by the hospital resuscitation team and spontaneous cardiac rhythm restarted after 20 minutes. She required continuous artificial ventilation and was unconscious for a week. Over the next six weeks she gradually regained consciousness but could not be weaned from the ventilator. She was tetraplegic—presumably as a result of spinal cord damage from hypoxia—but regained some weak finger movements over two months. At three months her improvement had tailed off and she was virtually paralysed in all four limbs and dependent on the ventilator. She died five months after the cardiac arrest. She was supported throughout her illness by her devoted and intelligent husband, who left his work to be with her and continued to hope for a spontaneous cure until very near the end.

Importance of clinical judgment

We are fortunate indeed that there appears to be greater understanding between patient and doctor in the UK, as reflected by the much lower incidence of medicolegal activity. Nevertheless, we must take heed of experience from across the Atlantic. The need is clear for us to ensure that futile attempts at resuscitation are minimised and that the modern medical profession does not get a name for prolonging misery and the process of dying simply because we are afraid to make a decision or because we are too proud to admit that all patients die sometime and that that time may be imminent.

On occasions, the decision whether or not to resuscitate may be fudged by the clinician. "Try just a bit and see if he responds" is fraught with danger and is more likely to prolong the vegetative and dying process. Nevertheless, the decision not to resuscitate should not be confused with other treatment destined to make the patient comfortable and enable him to take his chance if fate so decrees. Clinical judgment here is of the essence.

1 Wildsmith JAW, Dennyson WG, Myers KW. Results of resuscitation following cardiac arrest. *Br J Anaesth* 1972;44:716–9.
2 Eltringham RJ, Baskett PJF. Experience with a hospital resuscitation service including an analysis of 258 calls to patients with cardiorespiratory arrest. *Resuscitation* 1973;2:57–68.
3 Hershey CO, Fisher L. Why outcome of cardiopulmonary resuscitation in general wards is so poor. *Lancet* 1982;ii:32.
4 Sowden GR, Baskett PJF, Robins DW. Factors associated with survival and eventual cerebral status following cardiac arrest. *Anaesthesia* 1984;39:1.
5 De Bard ML. Cardiopulmonary resuscitation: analysis of six years experience and review of the literature. *Ann Emerg Med* 1981;10:408–16.
6 McPhail A, Moore S, O'Connor J, Woodward C. One hospital's experience with a "Do not resuscitate" policy. *Can Med Assoc J* 1981;125:830–6.
7 Canadian Medical Association. *Proceedings of the annual meeting including the transactions of the General Council 1974.* Ottawa: Canadian Medical Association, 1974.
8 Lo B, Steinbrook RL. Deciding whether to resuscitate. *Arch Intern Med* 1983;143:1561–3.

A 9 year old boy was admitted with 50% burns (mostly full thickness) of his face and head, chest, and arms. His nose and parts of his ears and most of his finger tips were destroyed. His corneas were opaque. He had also received severe thermal injury to his respiratory tract, requiring endotracheal intubation and artificial ventilation. At one stage his arterial Po_2 fell to 5·3 kPa (40 mm Hg) despite an inspired oxygen concentration of 80% and 7 cm H_2O positive end expiratory pressure. His devoted mother was divorced and had three other children. A decision was made to withhold dopamine and other resuscitative measures if they should be needed, but he improved spontaneously with the support of intravenous fluids and artificial ventilation. He and his family and friends face difficult times ahead.

FURTHER READING

Adgey AA. Electrical energy requirements for ventricular fibrillation. *Br Heart J* 1978; **40**: 1197–9.

American Heart Association. Standards and guidelines for cardiopulmonary resuscitation (CPR) and emergency cardiac care (ECC). *JAMA* 1980; **244**: 453–509.

American Heart Association. Standards and guidelines for cardiopulmonary resuscitation (CPR) and emergency cardiac care (ECC). *JAMA* 1986; **225**: 2905–92.

Babbs CF. New versus old theories of blood flow during CPR. *Crit Care Med* 1980; **8**: 191–5.

Baskett PJF. The need to disseminate knowledge of resuscitation into the community. *Anaesthesia* 1982; **37**: 74–6.

Baum RS, Alvarez H, Cobb LA. Survival after resuscitation from out of hospital ventricular fibrillation. *Circulation* 1974; **50**: 1231–5.

Bishop RL, Weisfeldt ML. Sodium bicarbonate administration during cardiac arrest. *JAMA* 1976; **235**: 506–9.

Bond W. Inactivation of hepatitis B virus by intermediate to high level disinfectant chemicals. *J Clin Microbiol* 1983; **18**: 535–8.

Broy RJ. The management of cardiac arrests in infants and children. *Br J Hosp Med* 1985; August: 72–81.

Caldwell G, Millar G, Quinn E, Vincent R. Simple mechanical methods for cardioversion. Defence of the precordial thump and cough version. *Br Med J* 1985; **291**: 627–30.

Casey W. CPR: A survey of standards among junior hospital doctors. *J R Soc Med* 1984; **77**: 921–2.

Chamberlain DA. Advanced life support. *Br Med J* 1989; **299**: 446–8.

Chandra N, Rudikoff M, Weisfelt M. Simultaneous chest compression and ventilation at high airway pressure during cardiopulmonary resuscitation. *Lancet* 1980; **i**: 175–8.

Crampton JA, Crampton RS, Sipes NJ, et al. Energy levels and patient weight in ventricular defibrillation. *JAMA* 1979; **242**: 1380.

Criley JM. CPR research 1960–1984: discoveries and advances. *Ann Emerg Med* 1984; **9**: 756–8.

Criley JM, Blaufuss AH, Kissel GL. Cough induced cardiac compression: self induced form of cardiopulmonary resuscitation. *JAMA* 1976; **236**: 1246–50.

Cummins RO, Eisenberg MS. Prehospital cardiopulmonary resuscitation. Is it effective? *JAMA* 1985; **253**: 2408–12.

Cummins RO, Eisenberg MS. CPR American style. *Br Med J* 1985; **291**: 1401–3.

Cummins RO, Schubach JA, Litwin PE, Hearne TR. Training lay persons to use automatic external defibrillators: success of initial training and one year retention of skills. *Am J Emerg Med* 1989; **7**: 143–9.

Eisenberg MS, Bergner L, Hallstrom AP. Cardiac resuscitation in the community: importance of rapid provision and implications for program planning. *JAMA* 1979; **241**: 1905–7.

Eisenberg MS, Copass MK, Hallstrom AP, et al. Treatment of out of hospital cardiac arrest with rapid defibrillation by emergency medical technicians. *N Engl J Med* 1980; **302**: 1379–83.

Eisenberg MS, Hallstrom AP, Carter WB, et al. Emergency CPR instruction via telephone. *Am J Public Health* 1985; **75**: 47–50.

Evans AL, Brody BA. The do not resuscitate order in teaching hospitals. *JAMA* 1985; **253**: 2236–9.

Fye WB. Ventricular fibrillation and defibrillation: historical perspectives with emphasis on the contributions of John MacWilliams, Carl Wiggers and William Kouwenhoven. *Circulation* 1985; **71**: 858–65.

Glaser MD, Nadler JP. Hepatitis B virus in a CPR course. *Arch Intern Med* 1985; **145**: 1653–5.

Greenberg MI. Endotracheal drugs state of the art. *Ann Emerg Med* 1984; **9**: 789–90.

Harrison EE, Amey BD. Use of calcium in electromechanical dissociation. *Ann Emerg Med* 1984; **13**: 844.

Hedges JR, Barsan WB, Doan LA, et al. Central versus peripheral intravenous routes in cardiopulmonary resuscitation. *Am J Emerg Med* 1984; **2**: 385–90.

Jones RH. Management of cardiac arrest in the community. A survey of resuscitation services. *Br Med J* 1983; **287**: 968–71.

Kihn GJ, White BC, Swetnam RE, et al. Peripheral vs central circulation times during CPR. A pilot study. *Ann Emerg Med* 1981; **10**: 417–9.

Kouwenhoven WB, Jude JR, Knickerbocker GG. Closed chest cardiac massage. *JAMA* 1960; **173**: 1064–7.

Lo B, Saika G, Strill W, et al. "Do not resuscitate" decisions. A prospective study of three teaching hospitals. *Arch Intern Med* 1985; **145**: 1115–7.

Lund I, Skulberg A. Cardiopulmonary resuscitation by lay people. *Lancet* 1976; **ii**: 702–4.

McIntyre KM. Cardiopulmonary resuscitation and the ultimate coronary care unit. *JAMA* 1980; **244**: 510–11.

McKenna SP, Glendon AI. Occupational first aid training: decay in CPR skills. *Journal of Occupational Psychology* 1985; **58**: 109–17.

Maier GW, Tyson GS, Olsen CO, et al. The physiology of external cardiac massage: high impulse cardiopulmonary resuscitation. *Circulation* 1984; **70**: 86–101.

Mancini ME, Kaye W. The effect of time since training on house officers' retention of CPR skills. *Am J Emerg Med* 1985; **3**: 31–2.

Marsden A. Basic life support. *Br Med J* 1989; **299**: 442–5.

Marteau M, Johnston M, Wynne G, Evans TR. Cognitive factors in the explanation of the mismatch between confidence and competence in performing basic life support. *Psychology and Health* 1989; **3**: 173–82.

Melker R. Asynchronous and other alternative methods of ventilation during CPR. *Ann Emerg Med* 1984; **13**: 758–61.

Melker R. Recommendations for ventilation during cardiopulmonary resuscitation. Time for change? *Crit Care Med* 1985; **13**: 882–3.

Miller J, Tech D, Horivitz L, et al. The precordial thump. *Ann Emerg Med* 1984; **13**: 791–4.

Myerburg RJ, Estes D, Zaman L, et al. Outcome of resuscitation from bradyarrhythmic or asystolic prehospital cardiac arrest. *J Am Coll Cardiol* 1984; **4**: 1118.

Niemann JT, Criley JM, Rosborough JP, et al. Predictive indices of successful cardiac resuscitation after prolonged arrest and experimental cardiopulmonary resuscitation. *Ann Emerg Med* 1985; **14**: 521–8.

Niemann JT, Rosborough JP, Hausknecht M, et al. Cough CPR. Documentation of systemic perfusion in man and in an experimental model. A "window" to the mechanism of blood flow in external CPR. *Crit Care Med* 1980; **8**: 141–6.

Niemann JT, Rosborough JP, Ung S, et al. Haemodynamic effects of continuous abdominal binding during cardiac arrest and resuscitation. *Am J Cardiol* 1984; **53**: 269–74.

Oates S, Williams GL, Rees GAD. Cardiopulmonary resuscitation in late pregnancy. *Br Med J* 1988; **297**: 404–5.

Olsen DW, Thompson BM, Darin JC, et al. A randomized comparison study of bretyliumtosylate and lidocaine in resuscitation of patients from out of hospital ventricular fibrillation in a paramedic system. *Ann Emerg Med* 1984; **13**: 807–10.

Ornato JP, Gonzalez ER, Garnett AR, Levine RL, McUing BK. Effect of cardiopulmonary resuscitation compression rate on end-tidal carbon dioxide concentration and arterial pressure in man. *Crit Care Med* 1988; **16**: 241–5.

Partridge JF, Geddes JS. Cardiac arrest after myocardial infarction. *Lancet* 1966; **i**: 807–8.

Pennington JE, Taylor J, Lown B. Chest thump for reverting ventricular tachycardia. *N Engl J Med* 1970; **283**: 1192–5.

Redding JS. Effective routes of drug administration during cardiac arrest. *Anaesth Analg* 1967; **46**: 253–8.

Roberts JR, Greenberg MI, Knaub MA, et al. Blood levels following intravenous and endotracheal epinephrine administration. *JACEP* 1979; **8**: 53–6.

Roth R, Stewart RD, Rogers K, et al. Out of hospital cardiac arrest: factors associated with survival. *Ann Emerg Med* 1984; **1**: 237–43.

Royal College of Physicians. Resuscitation from cardiopulmonary arrest: training and organisation. *J R Coll Physicians Lond* 1987; **21**: 1–8.

Rudikoff MT, Maughan WL, Eftron M, et al. Mechanism of blood flow during cardiopulmonary resuscitation. *Circulation* 1980; **61**: 345–52.

Ruskin JN. Automatic external defibrillators and sudden cardiac arrest. *N Engl J Med* 1988; **319**: 713–5.

Safar P. Ventilatory efficacy of mouth to mouth artificial respiration. Airway obstruction during manual and mouth to mouth artificial respiration. *JAMA* 1958; **167**: 335–41.

Safar P, Bircher NS. Cardiopulmonary cerebral resuscitation. London: WB Saunders, 1988.

Safar P, Escarrago L, Change F. A study of upper airway obstruction in the unconscious patient. *J Appl Physiol* 1959; **14**: 760–4.

Sanders AB, Harvey MO. The physiology of cardiopulmonary resuscitation—an update. *JAMA* 1984; **252**: 3283–5.

Skinner DV. CPR skills of preregistration house officers. *Br Med J* 1985; **290**: 1549–50.

Stueven HA, Thompson BM, Aprahamian C, et al. Calcium chloride reassessment of use in astystole. *Ann Emerg Med* 1984; **13**: 820.

Tacker GJ. Importance of prolonged compression during CPR in man. *N Engl J Med* 1977; **296**: 1515–7.

Taylor AE, Guyton AC, Bishop VS. Permeability of the alveolar membrane to solutes. *Circ Res* 1965; **16**: 353–62.

Thompson RG, Hallstrom AP, Cobb LA. Bystander initiated cardiopulmonary resuscitation in the management of ventricular fibrillation. *Ann Intern Med* 1979; **90**: 737–40.

Tweed WA, Bristow G, Doner N. Resuscitation from cardiac arrest. Assessment of a system providing only basic life support outside of hospital. *Can Med Assoc J* 1980; **122**: 297–300.

Walters G, Glucksman E. Retention of skills by advanced trained ambulance staff. Implications for monitoring and retraining. *Br Med J* 1989; **298**: 649–50.

Weaver FJ, Ramirez AG, Dorfman SB, Raizner AE. Trainees' retention of CPR. How quickly they forget. *JAMA* 1979; **241**: 901–3.

Weaver WD, Cobb LA, Copass MK, et al. Ventricular defibrillation. A comparative trial using 175 J and 320 J shocks. *N Engl J Med* 1982; **307**: 1101–6.

Weaver WD, Copass MK, Bufi D, et al. Improved neurologic recovery and survival after early defibrillation. *Circulation* 1984; **69**: 943–8.

Weaver WD, Copass MK, Cobb LA, et al. A new compact automatic external defibrillator designed for lay person use. *J Am Coll Cardiol* 1985; **5**: 457.

Weaver WD, Hill D, Fahrenbruch CE, et al. Use of the automatic external defibrillator in the management of out of hospital cardiac arrest. *N Engl J Med* 1988; **319**: 661–6.

Wei JY, Green HL, Weisfeldt ML. Cough facilitated cardioversion of ventricular tachycardia. *Am J Cardiol* 1980; **45**: 174–6.

Wright D, James C, Marsden AK, Mackintosh AF. Defibrillation by ambulance staff who had extended training. *Br Med J* 1989; **299**: 96–7.

Zoll PM, Zoll RH, Falk RH, et al. External non-invasive temporary cardiac pacing clinical trials. *Circulation* 1985; **71**: 937–44.

Index

ABC of resuscitation   1
Abdominal binders   13
Abdominal haemorrhage   28, 29, 32
Abdominal thrusts   2, 13, 57
  manikins   46
Acid base balance   38–39
Accident and Emergency Departments   37
  cleaning up   29
  "debriefing"   29
  equipment   26
  megacode   27, 42, 47, 49
  relatives' room   29
  resuscitation area   26
  resuscitation scheme   27–9
  transfer of responsibility   29
  use of resuscitation room   29
Acidaemia   9
Acidosis   7, 10, 38, 52
Actronics (USA)   49
Adam Rouilly Ltd (UK)
  address   49
  manikins   46
Adjuncts See Airway adjuncts
Adrenaline   8, 9, 11, 20, 60
  prefilled syringes   20
  pregnancy   52
Adult respiratory distress syndrome   64
Advanced life support
  general practice   17–20
  infants and children   59–61
  manikins   47–48
  training   40, 42, 43, 45
Advanced trauma life support
  airway care   31
  circulation   32
  cricothyroidotomy   31
  monitoring   33
  neurological assessment   32
  oxygenation and ventilation   31–32
  scheme   30
  spinal injuries   30
After care See Postresuscitation care
AIDS   4, 65
Airway   27, 31, 62
  contamination   13
  establishing   1–2
  infants and children   57–8, 59
  isolation   16
  manikins   46
  patency   12–14
  pregnancy   51
  support   15–16
Airway adjuncts   4, 15–16, 65
  infants and children   59
Airway, obstructed   27
  at birth   55
  causes   1, 12, 31
  infants and children   57
  suction clearance   13, 27, 31
  surgical intervention   14, 27, 31
  treatment   2, 12, 13
Alcohol   29, 62
Alderson Research Laboratories Inc (USA)
  address   49
  manikins   46
Alpha adrenergic stimulation   9
Ambu International UK Ltd   47
  ABC model   46
  address   49
  intubation trainer   48
  "Man"   46
  manikins   46
Ambulance crews   18
  audit   24
  drugs used   23
  emergencies handled   24
  retraining   23
  training   22, 23, 24, 53

Ambulances, resuscitation
  benefits   24
  coordination   24
  equipment   24
  future   21
  general practitioners   25
  successful resuscitations   24
  United Kingdom   22
  United States of America   21
American College of Surgeons   30
American Heart Association   41, 45, 46
Anaesthesia   52
Anaphylactic shock drug kit   20
Anoxia   9, 53
Antepartum haemorrhage   19
Antibiotics   64
Antishock trousers   28, 32
Antitetanus immunoglobulin   29
Aortic aneurysms   28
Apnoea   27, 31, 37
  near drowning   62, 63
  pregnancy   53
Arrhythmias   5, 6, 18, 63
  simulation   48
Arterial catheterisation   39
Asphyxia   13, 62
Aspiration pneumonia   1
Aspirin   18
Assessment of patient   1
Asthma   10, 19
Asystole   5, 7, 18, 19
  after defibrillation   8
  birth   56
  causes   9
  diagnosis   9
  management   9–10
Atrioventricular block   10
Atrioventricular node   9
Atropine   9, 52, 60
  prefilled syringes   20
Audit   24
Autonomic nervous system   10
AVPU mnemonic   32
Ayres T piece, modified   59

Back blows   2, 13
  infants and children   57
  manikins   46
Bag mask ventilation   16, 27, 32, 41, 51, 63
  infants and children   59
  manikins   47
Barbiturate coma   38, 64
Basic life support   1–4, 7
  confidence and competence   42
  hospital staff   34, 35
  infants and children   57–8
  manikins   46–7
  pregnancy   51–2
  skill retention   41, 53
  training   17, 40, 42, 43, 44, 45
Beta stimulation   11
Birth
  equipment   54
  high risk deliveries   54
  preterm resuscitation   56
  procedure at delivery   55
  resuscitation procedure   55
Birthweight   61
Blood
  body fluids   65
  culture   63, 64
  gases   27, 33, 38, 39, 52, 61, 63
  group O   32
  loss   32
  samples   28
  sugar   61
  transfusion   28
  volume restoration   19

Blood pressure   29, 33, 39, 61
  cuffs for infants   60
Body fluids   65
Body weight, paediatric   61
Brachial pulse   58
Bradycardia   18, 52
  infants and children   58
  newborn   56
Brain See also Cerebral
  blood flow to   8
  glucose   37
  ischaemia   37, 38
  microthrombus formation   37
Brain damage   5, 62, 64
  failure of reperfusion   37
  minimising   38
  pregnancy   53
Breathing   2, 27–8, 31, 62
  birth   55
  infants and children   57, 58, 59
  postresuscitation   38
  pregnancy   51
Bretylium tosylate   8, 52
Brighton experiment   22, 23
British Association for Immediate Care
  (BASICS)   19
  address   20
British Heart Foundation   18, 20
Bronchial intubation   16, 28, 39
Brook airway   15
Brunswick Manufacturing Co Inc (USA)   49
Bupivicaine toxicity   52
Burns   28

Caesarean section   53
Calcium administration   10, 11, 37
Calcium antagonists   11, 37
Calcium chloride   60
Canadian Medical Association   67
Cannulae, intravenous   60
Carbon dioxide
  cerebrospinal fluid   38
  partial pressure   27, 37, 38
Cardiac arrest   1, 32, 62
  general practice   17–20
  hypovolaemia   28
  infants and children   57
  management   5–8, 9–10, 11
  mechanisms   9
  megacode   27, 42, 47, 49
  mortality   17
  pregnancy   50
  simulated   42
  successful resuscitation   37
  team   35
Cardiac massage in newborn   56
Cardiac output   37, 38
Cardiac pacing   10, 11
Cardiac rhythm
  infants and children   60
  simulation   48
Cardiac tamponade   10, 11
  diagnosis   39
Cardiff resuscitation wedge   51
Cardiopulmonary resuscitation   1–4
  bystander   25, 35
  caesarean section   53
  house officers' inability   40
  near drowning   62, 63
  one rescuer   3, 40
  posters   42
  quality of training   44
  two rescuers   4
Carotid pulse   3, 37, 63
  manikins   47
Catheterisation
  arterial   39
  intravenous   32

Catheterisation—cont.
pulmonary 39
umbilical vein 56
urinary 29, 33, 39
Centers for Disease Control 65
Central venous pressure 29, 39, 61
Cerebral arteries 9
Cerebral blood flow 11, 37, 38
Cerebral oedema 37, 38, 64
Cerebral perfusion pressure 38
Cerebrospinal fluid 38
Cervical spine 1, 12
fractures 30
radiography 13, 27, 29, 30, 31, 61
stabilisation 13, 30
Chedoke and McMaster Hospitals, Hamilton,
Ontario, Canada 67
Chest
burns 28
drainage 28
injuries 12, 13, 27
pain 17, 18
radiography 27, 29, 39, 63
Chest compressions 7, 9, 13, 38, 39, 63
infants and children 58
manikins 47
pregnancy 51, 52
rate 3
technique 3
Children See Infants and children
Chin lift 2, 12, 31
Choanal atresia 55
Choking 2, 13–4
infants and children 57
manikins 46
Cholinergic activity 9
Circulation 3–4, 28, 32, 63
infants and children 58, 60
pregnancy 51
CLA (West Germany)
address 49
manikins 46, 48
Coma scales 29
Glasgow 32, 33
Community role 25
Compression: ventilation ratios 3, 4, 51
infants and children 58
newborn 56
Computer technology 49
Consciousness levels 29, 32
Contagious diseases 35
Convulsions 29
Coronary arteries 9
disease 5
Corticosteroids 28
Costochondral dislocation 38
Coughing 2, 13
Counterpulsation 13
Cricoid pressure manoeuvre 13, 51
Cricothyroidotomy 14, 27, 31
Croup 58
Cyclizine 20

Dangers of resuscitation 4
Death See Sudden death
Defibrillation
guidelines 7
infants and children 60
maximum number of shocks 8
pregnancy 52
principle 6
procedure 7
shock sequence 7
training 7, 48
Defibrillators 6, 60
advisory 6, 18, 20, 23
ambulances 18
automatic 6–7
general practice 17, 20
Delivery See Birth
Department of Health (and Social
Security) 22, 23, 24
Dextrose 8, 60

Diamorphine 18
dosage 20
Diaphragmatic hernia 13, 56
Diazepam 29
Digoxin 39
Diuretics 39
Dopamine 60
Drowning and near drowning 28
clinical features 62
definition 62
field management 62–3
hospital management 63
incidence 62
late complications 64
Drug administration
advanced cardiac life support 20
ambulance crews 23
defibrillation 8, 18, 52
infants and children 60–1
newborn 56
pregnancy 52
Dual-Aid airway 15
Dual response to chest pain 18, 19, 20

Echocardiogram 39
Electrical defibrillation See Defibrillation
Electrocardiogram 29, 33, 60
asystole 9
electromechanical dissociation 11
monitoring 39
simulated 48
ventricular fibrillation 5, 6, 7
Electrode jelly 6, 8
Electrodes 6
adhesive 7
paediatric 60
positions 6, 8
Electrolytes 38, 61, 63
abnormalities 9, 10
Electromechanical dissociation 18, 37
causes 10, 19, 39
experimental 10
fluid loss 19
management 11
Emphysema 28
End point of resuscitation 37
Endotracheal tubes for infants and
children 59
Epidural anaesthesia 52
Epiglottis 16
Epileptic fits 38
Equipment
accident and emergency departments 26
general practice 19
paediatric 60
resuscitation at birth 54
Escharotomy 28
Ethics 35
clinical judgment 67
decisions 66
formal policies 67
inappropriate resuscitation 66
Expiration, obstructed 15
Expired air respiration 14–5, 35
infants and children 58
manikins 47
pregnancy 51
technique 3
user acceptance 41-2

Face mask 42, 47
resuscitation at birth 55, 56
Femoral pulse 3
Femoral vein 60
Fetus
heart beat 56
hypoxia 53
Fever 64
Finger sweeps 2, 57
First aiders 41
Flail segment 28, 31, 38
Fluid
ingestion 13

loss 19
overload 60
replacement 19, 32
Food ingestion 13
Foreign bodies 1, 2, 13, 51, 57, 62
Fractures 29
cervical spine 30
rib 38
Frenchay Hospital, Bristol 67
Frusemide 60

Gag reflex 38
Gastric See Stomach
Gastroenteritis 57, 60
Gaumard Scientific Company Inc (USA)
address 49
manikins 46
Gel pads 6
General practice
cardiovascular emergencies 17–8
equipment 19–20
hypovolaemia 19
respiratory emergencies 19
General practitioners
ambulance crews 25
life support skills 17
Glasgow coma scale 32, 33
Glucose 39
cerebral 37
Gram negative organisms 64
Guedel airway 15, 59, 63

Haemodynamics, post resuscitation 39
Haemorrhage 27
antepartum 19
intraventricular 54
shock 28, 32
Head injuries 13
Head tilt 2, 12, 31
Head's paradoxical reflex 55
Heart See also Cardiac
congenital disease 57
failure 5
normal beat 5
thrombus 10
tumour 10
Heart rate
infants and children 58, 60
newborn 55, 56
Heartsim 2000 rhythm simulator 48
Heimlich's manoeuvre 2, 13
Hepatitis B virus 65
Hiatus hernia 13
Hilt-way airway 15
Hospitals 40
areas 34
basic life support 34, 35
cardiac arrest team 35
discharge rates 35, 66
manikin provision 49
near drowning 63
resuscitation panel 35
resuscitation training officer 36
Human immunodeficiency virus (HIV) 55,
56, 65
Hypercalcaemia 11
Hyperkalaemia 9, 11
Hypertension 39
Hyperventilation, mechanical 7, 29, 37, 38,
60, 64
Hypocalcaemia 11
Hypoglycaemia 29
Hypokalaemia 39
Hypotension 18, 32
Hypothermia 38, 61, 62, 63
Hypovolaemia 10, 11, 28, 32
infants and children 57, 60
Hypoxia 7, 10, 19, 37, 53, 57, 62, 63, 64
preterm intubation 56

Infants and children
advanced life support 59–61
basic life support 57–8

body weight 61
mortality 57
postresuscitation care 61
resuscitation chart 61
temperature 61
Infections
risk 15, 45, 47, 65
upper airway 58
Inferior vena caval compression 50
relief 51, 53
Injuries
head 13
multiple 29, 30–3
penetrating 28
Insulin 39
Intensive care
areas in hospital 34
unit 37
Intermittent positive pressure ventilation 14
International Medication Systems 20
Intestinal obstruction 13
Intracranial haematoma 29
Intracranial pressure 29, 64
monitoring 38
Intravenous infusion 19, 32
infants and children 60
manikins 48
sites 28
Intraventricular haemorrhage 56
Intubation See Tracheal intubation
Ischaemia
cerebral 37, 38
myocardial 5
Ischaemic heart disease 5
Isoprenaline 11, 60

Jaw thrust 12, 31
Jet ventilation 14, 31
Joint Colleges Ambulance Liaison
Committee 24
Jugular veins 28, 60

Koker Resim (Japan) 49

Lactic acid 38
Laerdal Medical (UK) Ltd
address 15, 49
infusion arm 48
intubation trainers 48
manikins 46
pocket mask and valve 15
rhythm simulator 48
Laryngeal mask airway 16
Laryngeal oedema 31, 50
Laryngoscopy 13, 16
at birth 55, 56
infants and children 59
pregnancy 52
Laryngotomy 14, 27, 31
Leg haemorrhage 28, 32
Life support See Advanced life support;
Advanced trauma life support; basic life
support
Lifeway 15
Lignocaine 8, 18, 39, 52, 60
prefilled syringes 20
Limb movements 29
"Logrolling" 13
Lungs
blast injuries 28
contusions 28, 31
water injury 62, 64

Manikins 36, 43, 51
advanced life support 47–8
basic life support 46
computerised 49
disinfection 45, 65
display of performance 49
distributors 49
evaluation of progress 49
hepatitis B 65

hospital provision 49
selection 45
Medical student training 43
Megacode scheme 27, 42, 49
manikin 47
Mannitol 29
Maternal mortality 50
Meconium aspiration 56
Methoxamine 11
Methylprednisolone 28
Metoclopramide 20
Microthrombus formation, cerebral 37
Miller Report 23
Monitoring 29, 33
Morphine 18
dosage 20
Mouth to mask resuscitation 16, 32, 41, 63
manikins 47
pregnancy 51, 52
user acceptance 42
Mouth to mouth resuscitation 14, 63, 65
pregnancy 51, 52
user acceptance 41–2
Mouth to nose resuscitation 15, 51
manikins 47
Multiple injuries 29, 30–3
Myocardial infarction 5, 9, 10, 25
deaths 17
general practice 17–8
Myocardium 9
cell depolarisation 6
ischaemia 5
pump failure 10
rupture 10

Naloxone 20, 56
Nares, flaring 58
Nasal airway obstruction 12
Nasal resistance 15
NASCO (USA)
address 49
model 48
Nasogastric tubes 39
Nasopharyngeal tubes 15, 27, 31, 59
Nasotracheal intubation 31
National Health Service Training
Authority 24
course 23
National Staff Committee for Ambulance
Staff 23, 24, 25
Nebulisers 19
Neck
burns 28
immobilisation 13, 27, 30
lift 12
pregnancy 52
Needlestick injuries 65
Neurological assessment 29, 32
Neutropenia 64
Newborn
cardiac massage 56
core temperature 54
Nurse training 36, 42, 43

Obesity 13
Oesophagus
cardiac pacing 10
obturators 16
Opiate sedation, maternal 56
Oropharyngeal tubes 27, 31
Orotracheal intubation 31
Oropharynx
stimulation 15
suction clearance 14
Oscilloscope 6
"recovery" 7
simulated 48
Oxygen 10
consumption in pregnancy 50, 51
partial pressure 27, 38
saturation 29
Oxygenation 31, 38
after immersion 62, 63

Paddles, defibrillation See Electrodes
Paediatric resuscitation chart 61
Paramedical personnel 34
See also Ambulance crews
Pelvis
haemorrhage 28, 32
radiography 29
Peptic ulcer 19
Pericardial effusion 11
Peritoneal lavage 29
pH 38, 61
central monitoring 39
Pharyngeal suction 55
Pierre Robin syndrome 55
Plasma expansion 63
Pleural effusion 56
Pneumonia, aspiration 1
Pneumonitis, chemical 13
Pneumothorax 39, 56
tension 10, 11, 29, 31
traumatic 28, 31
Positive end expiratory pressure 64
Posters 42
Postresuscitation care
acid base balance 38–9
brain damage 37–8
cardiac output 37, 38, 39
checklist 38
haemodynamics 39
infants and children 61
respiration 38
Potassium, serum 38, 39
Precordial thump 7
Pregnancy 13
acute causes of death 50
advanced life support 52
basic life support 51-52
caesarean section 53
changes and resuscitation 50
training 53
Preterm resuscitation 56
Prochlorperazine 20
Pulmonary catheterisation 39
Pulmonary embolism 10, 11
Pulmonary oedema 64
Pulse 29, 33
brachial 58
carotid 3, 37, 47, 58
defibrillation 7,8
femoral 3, 58
haemorrhagic shock 32
Pupillary responses 29, 32
postresuscitation 39

Radiography 13, 27, 29, 30, 39, 61, 63
Recording Resusci Anne 46
Recovery positions 1, 12
manikins 46
Regional Ambulance Officers Group 24
Regurgitation 3, 13
pregnancy 51
Renal failure 39
Rendell-Baker mask 59
Respiratory arrest 62
Respiratory inadequacy 27
traumatic causes 31
Respiratory rate 29, 31, 33
Resusci Baby 46
Resusci Junior 46
Resuscitation Council of the United
Kingdom 7, 20, 40, 52
Resuscitation panel 35
Rewarming 63
Rib fractures 38
Road accidents 19
Royal College of Physicians: Report, 35, 40
Royal College of Surgeons of Edinburgh 17
Royal College of Surgeons of England 30

Safar S airway 15
Safar's triple manoeuvre 12
Saline solution 32
Salivary transmission of HIV 65

San Arena (P Burtscher) Switzerland
   address 49
   computerised simulators 49
   manikins 46
Saphenous vein 28
Seal Easy/Vent Easy mask-airway 15
Seattle, Washington 17, 35
   Medic 1 scheme 21
Sellick's manoeuvre 13
Septicaemia 57, 64
Shock
   anaphylactic 20
   cardiogenic 5
   early fluid replacement 19
   management 28, 32
Sim I manikin 49
Simulaids Inc (USA)
   address 49
   manikins 46
Sinus node 9, 10
Skillmeter Resusci Anne 46
Skull 29
Smoke inhalation 28
Sodium bicarbonate 8, 37, 38, 39, 52, 60, 63
   newborn 56
Spinal anaesthesia 52
Spinal cord lesions 27
Spinal injuries 13, 30
Sternal dislocation 38
Steroids 28, 38, 64
Stomach 16
   distension 3, 13, 39
   full 12
   inflation 13, 15
Subclavian vein 60
Suction 13, 27, 31, 51
   at birth 55, 56
   catheters 14, 59
   pumps 14
Sudden death 5
   asthma 19
   outside hospital 21
Sudden infant death syndrome 57
Survival rates 66
Sussex valve airway 15

Tachycardia See Ventricular tachycardia
Temperature, body 63
   infants and children 61
   newborn 54
Tension pneumothorax 10, 11, 28, 31
   relief 32
Tetanus prophylaxis 29
Thoracentesis 32
Thoracotomy 28
Throat 13
Thrombolytic agents 18
   prehospital use 25
Tongue supports 15, 27, 31
Tracheal intubation 12, 27, 31, 38, 63
   at birth 55, 56
   infants and children 59
   manikins 48
   pregnancy 51, 52
   risks 16
   technique 16
   unrecognised 16
Trachesostomy 14, 27
Training See also Manikins
   advanced life support 40, 42, 43
   ambulance crews 22, 23, 24
   basic life support 40, 42, 43
   better teaching 40
   confidence and competence 42
   defibrillation 7
   future developments 49
   general practitioners 25
   hospital staff 36, 40
   medical students 43
   nurses 36, 42, 43
   obstetric care staff 53
   recommendations 44
   skill expectation 45
   skill retention 36, 41–2, 53
   teaching methods 43
   team skills 49
Transcutaneous pacing 10
Transthoracic pacing 10
Transvenous ventricular pacing 10
Trauma 60
   See also Advanced trauma life support
Trendelenburg tilt 13

Ultrasound diagnostic 29
Umbilical vein catheterisation 56
Unconscious patient 1, 2, 12, 16, 31
   haemorrhage 32
   resuscitation scheme 27–9
Urinary catheterisation 29, 33, 39
Urine output 29, 33, 39
Uterus, gravid 50
   manual displacement 51

Vasopressor drugs 7, 11
Vasospasm, cerebral 37
Venous access 19, 23, 32
   infants and children 60
   manikins 48
Venous return in pregnancy 50, 51
Ventilation 27, 31–2, 61, 63
   elective 37–8
   infants and children 58, 59
   jet 31
   newborn 55
   pregnancy 51
Ventilation devices 15–6, 65
   neonatal 55
Ventilation masks 15–6, 42, 55
   paediatric 59
Ventilatory failure 28
Ventricular fibrillation 9, 10, 18, 23, 39, 52, 60
   definition 5
   defibrillation 5–7 8
   drug administration 8
   hypothermia 63
   loss of consciousness 5
   recurrence 8
   spontaneous remission 5
Ventricular tachycardia 7, 18, 52, 60
Viruses 65
Vitalograph Ltd (UK)
   address 49
   intubation trainer 48
Vomiting 3, 13, 15 16, 39
   after immersion 62, 63

White cell count 62